Yoga Fusion: Bridging Tradition, Science, and Modern Practice

Susanne J. Katts

Trademarks:

All trademarks, service marks, and trade names are the property of their respective owners and are used for identification purposes only. This book is not sponsored or endorsed by, or otherwise affiliated with, any of the organizations or individuals mentioned herein.

"Yoga Fusion: Bridging Tradition, Science, and Modern Practice"

Preface

Welcome to "Yoga Fusion: Bridging Tradition, Science, and Modern Practice." As both a seasoned yogi and a curious explorer of the human body and mind, I have always been fascinated by the intricate dance between ancient wisdom and modern science. This book is born out of a deep desire to bring these two worlds together, offering a comprehensive guide that honors the rich traditions of yoga while embracing the insights provided by contemporary scientific research.

Yoga has long been revered for its ability to transform lives, fostering physical health, mental clarity, and spiritual growth. Yet, for many, the practice of yoga remains shrouded in mystery and myth. In "Yoga Fusion," I aim to demystify yoga, presenting it as a practice that is accessible, scientifically validated, and profoundly beneficial for individuals of all backgrounds and abilities.

This book is structured to take you on a journey through the multifaceted world of yoga. We begin by acknowledging the diversity of human bodies and the importance of tailoring yoga practices to meet individual needs. You'll find practical advice on modifying poses for different anatomical structures and health conditions, ensuring that your practice is safe, effective, and uniquely yours.

As we move forward, we delve into the long-term effects of yoga, supported by robust scientific evidence. You'll discover how yoga can alleviate mental health challenges such as anxiety and depression, enhance cognitive function, and promote overall physical health. Comparative analyses with other forms of exercise underscore yoga's unique contributions to well-being.

Safety is paramount in any physical practice, and yoga is no exception. In the sections dedicated to safety and injury prevention, you'll learn how to identify high-risk poses, implement injury-prevention techniques, and maintain proper alignment. Expert insights from physiotherapists and experienced instructors provide a solid foundation for a safe practice.

Inclusivity is a core value in "Yoga Fusion." Special chapters address the needs of pregnant women, the elderly, and individuals with disabilities, offering adaptive techniques and inclusive practices. Through personal stories and expert advice, these sections highlight the transformative power of yoga for everyone.

The scientific research underpinning yoga is both fascinating and essential for informed practice. I provide a critical analysis of current studies, debunk common myths, and offer guidance on discerning credible information. This evidence-based approach empowers you to make informed decisions about your practice.

Holistic health is another key theme of this book. Integrating yoga with nutrition, meditation, and traditional medical treatments can significantly enhance your well-being. You'll find practical tips, case studies, and expert interviews that illustrate the benefits of a holistic approach.

Yoga's diversity is one of its greatest strengths. In exploring various styles of yoga, you'll gain insights into their unique characteristics and benefits, helping you choose the right style for your goals. Whether you're drawn to the foundational practices of Hatha yoga, the dynamic flow of Vinyasa, or the introspective nature of Yin yoga, there's something here for everyone.

Understanding yoga's cultural and historical roots enriches our practice and deepens our connection to this ancient art. You'll explore the origins of yoga, its evolution, and how modern practices honor tradition while embracing innovation.

For advanced practitioners, "Yoga Fusion" offers guidance on mastering complex poses, developing a personal practice, and continuing your growth. Inspirational stories from seasoned yogis and discussions on the spiritual and philosophical aspects of yoga encourage a lifelong journey of exploration and discovery.

This book is designed to be a comprehensive and accessible resource for yogis at every level. With detailed glossaries, additional resources, and contributions from experts, "Yoga Fusion" aims to be your trusted companion on the mat and beyond.

Thank you for embarking on this journey with me. May "Yoga Fusion" inspire, educate, and empower you to explore the depths of your practice, bridging tradition and science in your pursuit of holistic health and well-being.

Namaste,
Susanne J. Katts

Chapter 1: The Importance of Understanding Yoga from a Scientific and Practical Perspective

Yoga, often perceived as a timeless practice rooted in ancient traditions, is increasingly being studied through the lens of modern science. This chapter delves into why it is crucial to integrate both scientific and practical perspectives when approaching yoga.

Embracing Tradition with Modern Insight
Yoga's origins date back thousands of years, steeped in spiritual and philosophical traditions from ancient India. These traditions offer invaluable wisdom on the mind-body connection, holistic health, and spiritual growth. Understanding yoga's cultural and historical context provides a foundation for appreciating its depth and relevance in contemporary life.

Validating Yoga through Scientific Inquiry
In recent decades, scientific research has substantiated many of the anecdotal claims about yoga's benefits. Studies have shown that yoga can improve physical fitness, mental well-being, and even support medical treatments. By examining yoga through rigorous scientific methods, we can identify specific physiological changes, neurobiological effects, and psychological benefits associated with regular practice.

Holistic Approach to Well-being

Yoga's holistic approach addresses the interconnectedness of physical, mental, and emotional health. By practicing yoga, individuals not only enhance their flexibility and strength but also cultivate mindfulness, reduce stress, and improve overall quality of life. Scientific inquiry helps elucidate these multifaceted benefits, providing evidence-based strategies for integrating yoga into everyday life.

Enhancing Personal Practice
For practitioners, understanding the scientific principles underlying yoga can deepen their engagement and commitment to the practice. By knowing how yoga affects the body and mind on a physiological level, individuals can tailor their practice to achieve specific goals, address personal challenges, and maintain long-term well-being.

Bridging Tradition and Innovation
Integrating scientific insights with traditional teachings enriches the yoga experience. It encourages innovation while honoring the foundational principles that have sustained yoga for centuries. This synergy fosters a dynamic approach to yoga practice, welcoming new perspectives and evolving methodologies while preserving its essence.

Conclusion
This chapter sets the stage for exploring yoga through a dual lens of tradition and science. By appreciating yoga's ancient roots and embracing contemporary research, practitioners can cultivate a balanced and informed approach to their practice, unlocking its full potential for physical, mental, and spiritual growth.

In the chapters to come, we will delve deeper into specific aspects of yoga, examining how scientific understanding enhances each facet of practice. Join me on this journey to explore the transformative power of yoga from both ancient wisdom and modern insights.

Chapter 2: Individual Differences in Yoga Practice

Yoga is a deeply personal journey, influenced by the unique characteristics of each individual's body, mind, and lifestyle. This chapter explores the importance of recognizing and accommodating these differences to optimize the practice of yoga for every practitioner.

Understanding Body Types and Their Impact
No two bodies are alike, and each person brings a distinct anatomical structure to their yoga practice. Understanding body types — such as skeletal proportions, muscle mass, and flexibility — helps tailor yoga poses to individual needs. This awareness promotes safe alignment, prevents injury, and enhances the effectiveness of each posture.

Modifications for Different Anatomical Structures
Yoga poses can be modified to accommodate varying body structures and capabilities. By offering adjustments in alignment, props, or pose variations, practitioners can ensure accessibility and comfort without compromising the integrity of the pose. Case studies and practical examples illustrate how modifications cater to diverse body types and physical conditions.

Personalized Yoga Practices

Tailoring yoga practices to individual needs goes beyond physical adjustments — it encompasses personal goals, health considerations, and emotional well-being. Personalized yoga sequences can address specific challenges such as chronic pain, stress management, or enhancing athletic performance. Case studies highlight successful approaches to customizing yoga for optimal benefits.

Adapting Yoga for Specific Conditions
Yoga's adaptability extends to accommodating various health conditions, from arthritis to pregnancy. Specialized modifications and precautions ensure safety and efficacy, empowering individuals to engage in yoga as a therapeutic tool. Expert advice from healthcare professionals and experienced yoga instructors offers guidance on adapting poses to support overall well-being.

Conclusion
This chapter underscores the importance of recognizing and embracing individual differences in yoga practice. By tailoring yoga techniques to meet diverse needs and capabilities, practitioners can cultivate a sustainable and inclusive practice that fosters physical health, mental clarity, and personal growth.

In the following chapters, we will explore how these principles apply to specific aspects of yoga practice, from promoting mental health to advancing physical fitness. Join me as we navigate the diverse landscape of yoga, celebrating its transformative power in accommodating and embracing individual uniqueness.

Identifying Body Type: Understanding your body type involves recognizing your skeletal proportions, muscle flexibility, and overall mobility. A yoga instructor or physiotherapist can assess these factors and provide insights into how they might affect your practice. For example, someone with longer limbs might need adjustments in their stance or reach in certain poses compared to someone with shorter limbs.

Modifications for Anatomical Structures: Specific modifications depend on individual needs. For instance, if you have tight hips, using props like blocks or blankets can assist in achieving correct alignment in seated poses like Sukhasana (Easy Pose). Exploring different variations under the guidance of a qualified instructor ensures poses are adapted safely.

Personalizing Your Practice: Personalization involves aligning yoga practices with your goals and health considerations. Whether it's managing stress, improving flexibility, or recovering from injury, discussing these goals with an instructor allows them to tailor sessions or recommend suitable yoga styles like Restorative Yoga or Vinyasa Flow.

Adapting Yoga for Specific Conditions: Adapting yoga for conditions such as arthritis or pregnancy involves modifying poses to ensure comfort and safety. For example, individuals with arthritis might focus on gentle movements to enhance joint flexibility, while pregnant women benefit from prenatal yoga poses that support both mother and baby's well-being.

Safety of Modifications: Ensuring modifications are safe involves understanding your body's limits and seeking guidance from a qualified instructor. They provide feedback on alignment and offer alternative poses to prevent strain or injury. Listening to your body and communicating any discomfort during practice helps adjust techniques accordingly.

Success Stories and Case Studies: Hearing about others' experiences with personalized yoga can inspire confidence. Many practitioners share how tailored practices helped them achieve physical and mental wellness goals. Exploring testimonials or discussing with peers in yoga classes can provide further insights into the benefits of personalized approaches.

Role of Yoga Instructors: Instructors play a crucial role in guiding personalized practices. They assess your needs, provide hands-on adjustments, and suggest modifications tailored to your abilities. Their expertise ensures poses are adapted effectively, promoting progress and preventing potential injuries.

Balancing Tradition with Modern Adaptations: Yoga's adaptability embraces both traditional principles and modern adaptations. Integrating traditional poses with contemporary modifications allows for diverse practice approaches. Discussions with instructors or reading reputable yoga resources help strike this balance effectively.

Further Information and Resources: Seek reputable sources like yoga studios, certified instructors, or authoritative yoga publications for reliable information. Websites of established yoga organizations or books written by experienced yoga teachers often provide comprehensive guidance on adapting poses and practices.

Chapter 3: Anatomical Variations and Yoga

Yoga practice is deeply influenced by the anatomical variations present in every individual. This chapter delves into the importance of understanding these variations and how they impact the practice of yoga.

Embracing Individual Anatomy
Each person's anatomy, including bone structure, joint flexibility, and muscular strength, is unique. Recognizing these variations is essential for adapting yoga poses to suit different body types and abilities. By appreciating individual differences, practitioners can foster a more inclusive and effective yoga experience.

The Role of Skeletal Proportions
Skeletal proportions significantly influence how poses are performed. Longer limbs may require adjustments in stance or reach, while shorter limbs may affect balance and flexibility differently. Understanding these proportions helps in customizing poses for optimal alignment and safety.

Muscle Imbalances and Flexibility

Muscle imbalances, whether due to lifestyle, injury, or genetics, affect flexibility and range of motion in yoga poses. Addressing these imbalances through targeted stretches and strengthening exercises enhances pose stability and overall practice effectiveness. Case studies illustrate successful strategies for managing muscle asymmetry in yoga.

Joint Mobility and Yoga Poses
Joint mobility varies among individuals and impacts the depth and range of yoga poses. Some may naturally have greater flexibility in certain joints, while others require gradual adaptation to achieve optimal alignment. Techniques for improving joint mobility and safely expanding range of motion are explored in detail.

Adapting Poses for Physical Conditions
Anatomical variations also influence how yoga can be adapted for physical conditions such as scoliosis, hypermobility, or joint stiffness. Specialized modifications and props assist in achieving proper alignment and reducing strain. Expert advice from yoga therapists and medical professionals offers insights into tailored approaches for specific anatomical challenges.

Conclusion
This chapter underscores the significance of anatomical awareness in yoga practice. By acknowledging and accommodating individual anatomical variations, practitioners can cultivate a safe, personalized, and sustainable yoga practice that enhances physical well-being and fosters a deeper connection with the body.

In the subsequent chapters, we will explore how understanding anatomical variations informs the adaptation of yoga poses for specific health conditions, enhances pose precision, and promotes overall effectiveness in practice. Join me in uncovering the transformative potential of yoga through anatomical insight and personalized approach.

Chapter 3: Anatomical Variations and Yoga

Yoga practice is deeply influenced by the anatomical variations present in every individual. This chapter delves into the importance of understanding these variations and how they impact the practice of yoga.

Embracing Individual Anatomy
Each person's anatomy, including bone structure, joint flexibility, and muscular strength, is unique. Recognizing these variations is essential for adapting yoga poses to suit different body types and abilities. By appreciating individual differences, practitioners can foster a more inclusive and effective yoga experience.

The Role of Skeletal Proportions

Skeletal proportions significantly influence how poses are performed. Longer limbs may require adjustments in stance or reach, while shorter limbs may affect balance and flexibility differently. Understanding these proportions helps in customizing poses for optimal alignment and safety.

Muscle Imbalances and Flexibility
Muscle imbalances, whether due to lifestyle, injury, or genetics, affect flexibility and range of motion in yoga poses. Addressing these imbalances through targeted stretches and strengthening exercises enhances pose stability and overall practice effectiveness. Case studies illustrate successful strategies for managing muscle asymmetry in yoga.

Joint Mobility and Yoga Poses
Joint mobility varies among individuals and impacts the depth and range of yoga poses. Some may naturally have greater flexibility in certain joints, while others require gradual adaptation to achieve optimal alignment. Techniques for improving joint mobility and safely expanding range of motion are explored in detail.

Adapting Poses for Physical Conditions
Anatomical variations also influence how yoga can be adapted for physical conditions such as scoliosis, hypermobility, or joint stiffness. Specialized modifications and props assist in achieving proper alignment and reducing strain. Expert advice from yoga therapists and medical professionals offers insights into tailored approaches for specific anatomical challenges.

Conclusion

This chapter underscores the significance of anatomical awareness in yoga practice. By acknowledging and accommodating individual anatomical variations, practitioners can cultivate a safe, personalized, and sustainable yoga practice that enhances physical well-being and fosters a deeper connection with the body.

In the subsequent chapters, we will explore how understanding anatomical variations informs the adaptation of yoga poses for specific health conditions, enhances pose precision, and promotes overall effectiveness in practice. Join me in uncovering the transformative potential of yoga through anatomical insight and personalized approach.

Chapter 4: Understanding Body Types and Their Impact on Yoga Practice

Yoga is a highly individualized practice that can be profoundly influenced by each practitioner's unique body type. This chapter delves into the different body types and how they impact yoga practice, offering practical guidance on tailoring poses and sequences to enhance effectiveness and safety.

The Ectomorph, Mesomorph, and Endomorph Body Types

Understanding your body type can provide insights into how you approach yoga and which modifications might be beneficial.

Ectomorph: Characterized by a slim, linear physique with less muscle mass and fat. Ectomorphs typically have longer limbs and may find balance and strength-based poses more challenging. They benefit from focusing on building muscle strength and stability through poses like Plank and Warrior II.

Mesomorph: Known for a more muscular and athletic build, mesomorphs often have a natural aptitude for strength-based poses and dynamic sequences. They may excel in poses like Chaturanga and Chair Pose but should also incorporate flexibility and relaxation poses to ensure balanced practice.

Endomorph: Characterized by a higher percentage of body fat and a rounder physique, endomorphs may find flexibility and endurance-based poses more challenging. Gentle, supportive poses like Bridge and supported Restorative poses can enhance comfort and effectiveness.

Customizing Poses for Different Body Types
Each body type has its unique strengths and challenges. Here are some tailored strategies for modifying poses:

Ectomorphs:

Focus: Building strength and balance.
Modifications: Use props for support in balancing poses. Incorporate strength-building sequences.
Examples: Using blocks in Trikonasana (Triangle Pose) to enhance stability; incorporating weight-bearing poses like Downward Dog to build upper body strength.
Mesomorphs:

Focus: Flexibility and relaxation.
Modifications: Incorporate longer holds in flexibility poses, balance strength with stretching.
Examples: Deepening stretches in poses like Pigeon Pose to increase flexibility; integrating Yin Yoga to complement dynamic practice.
Endomorphs:

Focus: Flexibility, endurance, and comfort.
Modifications: Use props to enhance comfort, focus on breath and gentle movement.
Examples: Using bolsters in Supta Baddha Konasana (Reclined Bound Angle Pose) for support; incorporating gentle flow sequences to build endurance.
Practical Tips for All Body Types
Listen to Your Body: Pay attention to how your body feels in each pose. Avoid pushing into pain or discomfort.
Use Props: Props are not just for beginners. They can enhance alignment and support for any body type.
Personalize Your Practice: Tailor your yoga practice to your individual needs and goals. Consider working with a certified yoga instructor who can provide personalized guidance.
Balance Strength and Flexibility: Regardless of body type, a balanced practice that includes both strength-building and flexibility-enhancing poses promotes overall well-being.
Be Patient: Progress in yoga is gradual. Celebrate small milestones and be patient with your body's unique journey.
Conclusion
This chapter highlights the importance of understanding body types and their impact on yoga practice. By recognizing and embracing individual differences, practitioners can tailor their yoga experience to enhance safety, effectiveness, and personal growth.

In the following chapters, we will explore how to customize yoga practices for specific conditions and long-term benefits. Join me as we continue to delve into the intricacies of a personalized yoga journey, fostering a deeper connection between body, mind, and spirit.

Determining Your Body Type:

Response: Identifying your body type involves observing your physical characteristics. Ectomorphs tend to be slim with longer limbs, mesomorphs have a muscular and athletic build, and endomorphs have a rounder physique with a higher body fat percentage. Consulting with a fitness professional or yoga instructor can provide a more accurate assessment.
Recommended Poses for Each Body Type:

Response:

Ectomorphs: Focus on strength-building poses like Plank, Warrior II, and Downward Dog.
Mesomorphs: Balance strength with flexibility poses like Pigeon Pose, Forward Fold, and extended holds in dynamic sequences.
Endomorphs: Incorporate supportive and endurance-building poses like Bridge Pose, supported Restorative poses, and gentle flow sequences.
Modifying Poses for Your Body Type:

Response: Modifications depend on individual needs:
Ectomorphs: Use blocks in standing poses for balance; engage core muscles to stabilize.
Mesomorphs: Use straps to deepen stretches; focus on mindful transitions.
Endomorphs: Use bolsters and blankets for comfort in seated and supine poses; prioritize gentle movements.
Challenges and Advantages of Each Body Type:

Response:
Ectomorphs: Challenges with strength; advantages in flexibility.
Mesomorphs: Natural strength; need to work on flexibility and relaxation.
Endomorphs: Challenges with flexibility and endurance; advantages in poses requiring stability.
Balancing Strength and Flexibility:

Response: Incorporate a variety of poses in your practice:
Ectomorphs: Add strength-building sequences.
Mesomorphs: Include longer holds in flexibility poses.
Endomorphs: Mix gentle flow with supportive poses.
Role of Props:

Response: Props enhance alignment and support:
Ectomorphs: Blocks for balance.

Mesomorphs: Straps for deeper stretches.
Endomorphs: Bolsters and blankets for comfort.
General advice: Use props to achieve correct alignment and prevent strain.
Practicing Yoga Safely:

Response: Listen to your body and avoid pushing into pain. Use modifications and props to maintain alignment. Regularly consult with your instructor to ensure poses are adapted to your needs.
Body Type Changes Over Time:

Response: Body composition can change with regular practice. Adapt your yoga routine by reassessing your needs periodically, focusing on different aspects like strength, flexibility, or endurance as required.
Common Mistakes to Avoid:

Response:
Ectomorphs: Overstretching without building strength.
Mesomorphs: Neglecting flexibility and relaxation poses.
Endomorphs: Overexerting without adequate support.
General advice: Avoid comparing yourself to others; practice patience and consistency.
Finding a Qualified Yoga Instructor:

Response: Look for instructors with certifications from reputable yoga organizations. Attend trial classes to find an instructor who understands and respects your individual needs. Recommendations from other practitioners can also be valuable.

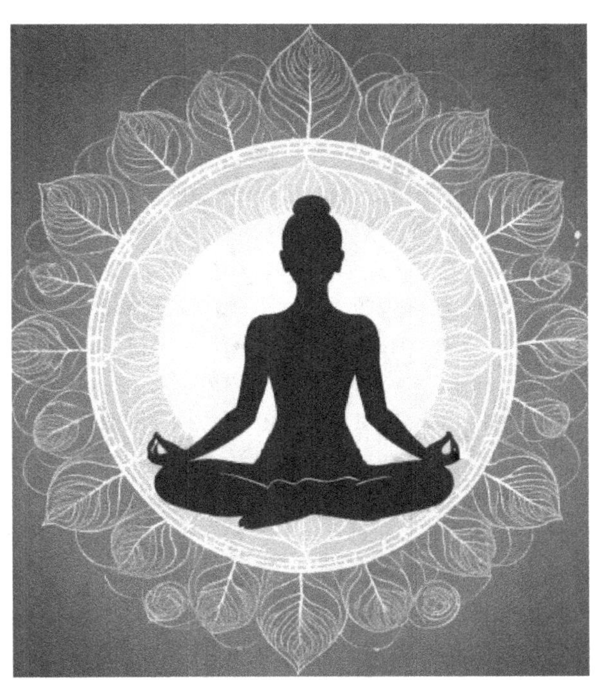

Chapter 5: Modifications for Different Anatomical Structures

Every individual's anatomy is unique, which means that standard yoga poses may not be suitable for everyone without modifications. This chapter focuses on practical strategies for adapting yoga poses to accommodate various anatomical structures, ensuring a safe and effective practice for all.

Understanding Anatomical Structures
Skeletal Structure: Variations in bone length, joint shape, and overall skeletal alignment can affect how poses are performed. Recognizing these differences is the first step in making appropriate modifications.
Muscle Composition: Muscle strength and flexibility vary widely among individuals, influencing how poses are approached and held.
Joint Mobility: The range of motion in joints can differ due to genetic factors, lifestyle, or injury. Understanding your joint mobility helps in adapting poses to prevent strain.
Common Anatomical Variations and Their Modifications
Long Limbs:

Challenges: Balance and alignment in poses.
Modifications: Use blocks in standing poses like Triangle (Trikonasana) to bring the ground closer and maintain stability. In seated forward bends, use straps to reach the feet comfortably.
Short Limbs:

Challenges: Reaching the floor or holding poses that require extended limbs.

Modifications: Use props like blocks and straps to extend reach. For example, in Forward Fold (Uttanasana), place hands on blocks instead of the floor.
Tight Hips:

Challenges: Difficulty in poses requiring hip flexibility, such as Pigeon Pose (Eka Pada Rajakapotasana).
Modifications: Use blankets or bolsters under the hips for support. Start with gentler hip openers like Bound Angle Pose (Baddha Konasana) and gradually progress.
Limited Shoulder Mobility:

Challenges: Poses that involve arm extension or overhead reaches, like Downward Dog (Adho Mukha Svanasana).
Modifications: Use straps to hold hands behind the back in poses like Cow Face Pose (Gomukhasana). Perform shoulder stretches regularly to increase mobility.
Back Issues:

Challenges: Performing backbends or twists without exacerbating pain.
Modifications: Use supportive poses like Bridge Pose (Setu Bandhasana) with a block under the sacrum. For twists, keep the spine long and twist gently, using props for support.
Knee Sensitivity:

Challenges: Poses that place pressure on the knees, such as Warrior Poses or Lotus Pose (Padmasana).
Modifications: Use padding under the knees in poses like Low Lunge (Anjaneyasana). Avoid deep knee bends and opt for gentler alternatives like Reclined Bound Angle Pose (Supta Baddha Konasana).
Using Props Effectively
Props are valuable tools for adapting poses to suit different anatomical structures. Here are some common props and their uses:

Blocks: Provide support and bring the ground closer in standing and seated poses.

Straps: Extend reach and maintain alignment in poses requiring flexibility.

Blankets: Offer cushioning and support in seated and kneeling poses.

Bolsters: Support the body in restorative poses, allowing for deeper relaxation.

Chairs: Assist in maintaining balance and support in standing poses.

Personalized Practice and Awareness

Listen to Your Body: Pay attention to signals of discomfort or pain and adjust accordingly. Practicing mindfulness ensures a safe and effective practice.

Work with an Instructor: A qualified yoga instructor can provide personalized guidance and adjustments to ensure poses are adapted correctly.

Progress Gradually: Allow time for your body to adapt to new modifications. Gradual progression reduces the risk of injury and enhances overall practice.

Conclusion

Understanding and respecting anatomical variations is crucial for a safe and effective yoga practice. By using modifications and props appropriately, practitioners can enhance their yoga experience, accommodating their unique anatomical structures. The next chapter will delve into how yoga can be tailored to address specific health conditions, further emphasizing the importance of personalized practice.

Identifying Your Own Anatomical Variations:

Response: Understanding your anatomical variations starts with self-awareness and observation. Pay attention to areas of discomfort or difficulty during your practice. Consulting with a qualified yoga instructor or physiotherapist can provide a professional assessment of your anatomical structure and help identify specific needs.

Specific Examples of Modifications:

Response:
Forward Fold (Uttanasana): Use blocks under hands to avoid straining the lower back.
Warrior I (Virabhadrasana I): Shorten the stance and use a chair for balance if you have limited hip mobility.
Seated Forward Bend (Paschimottanasana): Use a strap around your feet and a bolster under your knees for support.

Using Props Effectively:

Response: Props are essential tools in yoga to enhance comfort and alignment. Blocks can be used under hands or feet, straps help extend reach, blankets provide cushioning, bolsters support relaxation, and chairs assist in balance. Experiment with different props to find what works best for you in each pose.

Adaptable Yoga Styles:

Response: Restorative Yoga, Iyengar Yoga, and Hatha Yoga are particularly adaptable to anatomical variations. These styles emphasize alignment, use of props, and slower-paced movements, making them suitable for customized practice.

Addressing Discomfort or Pain in Modified Poses:

Response: If a modified pose causes discomfort, stop and reassess your alignment and prop usage. Ensure you're not pushing beyond your limits. Consult with an instructor to find an alternative modification or pose that suits your needs better.

Integrating Modifications in Group Classes:

Response: Communicate with your instructor before class about your need for modifications. Choose a spot where you feel comfortable making adjustments. Remember, modifications are a sign of a mindful and responsible practice, not a limitation.

Resources for Learning More About Anatomy and Yoga:

Response: Books like "The Key Muscles of Yoga" by Ray Long and "Yoga Anatomy" by Leslie Kaminoff and Amy Matthews are excellent resources. Online platforms like Yoga Journal and courses from Yoga Alliance provide valuable insights into anatomy and yoga.

Reassessing the Need for Modifications:

Response: Reassess your modifications periodically, especially as you progress in your practice. Regular check-ins with a yoga instructor can help you adjust your practice as your body changes and improves in strength and flexibility.

Combining Multiple Modifications in a Pose:

Response: Yes, you can combine modifications. For example, in Seated Forward Bend, use a strap around your feet and a bolster under your knees simultaneously. Ensure that combining modifications doesn't compromise your alignment or safety.

Common Mistakes to Avoid When Modifying Poses:

Response: Avoid pushing into pain, over-relying on props without proper alignment, and ignoring the body's feedback. Modifications should enhance the pose, not lead to strain or injury.
Finding a Qualified Yoga Instructor:

Response: Look for instructors certified by recognized yoga organizations like Yoga Alliance. Research their background and expertise in anatomy and therapeutic yoga. Attending workshops or private sessions can provide more personalized attention.
Advanced Modifications:

Response: Advanced modifications involve deeper engagement of muscles and refined alignment. For example, using a strap to bind hands in Gomukhasana (Cow Face Pose) or incorporating dynamic transitions between poses while maintaining modifications.
Enhancing Yoga Experience and Progression:

Response: Modifications allow you to practice poses safely and comfortably, leading to greater consistency and enjoyment. They help build strength and flexibility progressively, ensuring a sustainable and fulfilling yoga journey.
Role of Breathwork in Modified Poses:

Response: Breathwork, or pranayama, is crucial in yoga. It helps maintain focus, relaxes the body, and supports deeper engagement in poses. Practice deep, even breathing to enhance the benefits of modified poses.
Balancing Challenge and Respecting Limitations:

Response: Challenge yourself within your comfort zone. Use modifications to explore the edges of your abilities safely. Listen to your body's signals and avoid pushing into pain. Consistent practice with mindful progression leads to growth without injury.

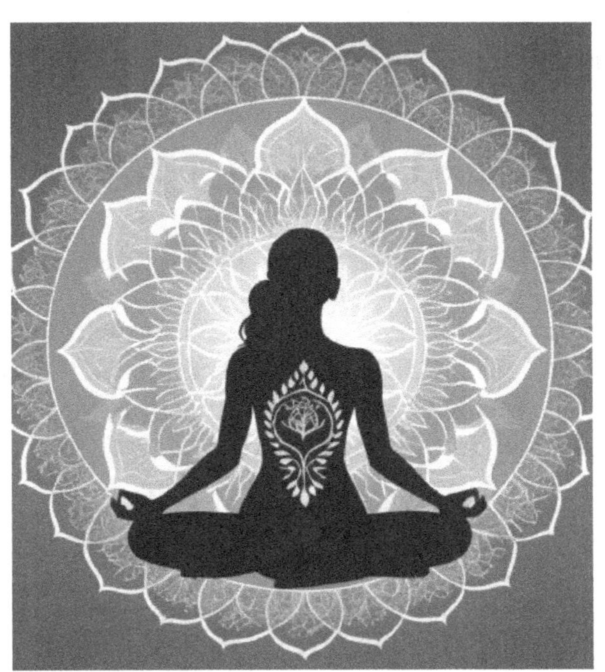

Chapter 6: Case Studies of Personalized Yoga Practices

This chapter delves into real-life examples of how personalized yoga practices have benefited individuals with different needs, anatomical structures, and health conditions. Through these case studies, readers can gain insights into the practical application of personalized modifications and the transformative impact of yoga tailored to individual requirements.

Case Study 1: Yoga for Back Pain Relief
Profile: Sarah, 45, Office Worker

Background: Sarah spends long hours at a desk, leading to chronic lower back pain. She has limited flexibility in her hamstrings and hip flexors.

Personalized Practice:

Assessment: Initial assessment revealed tight hamstrings and weak core muscles contributing to her back pain.
Modifications:
Forward Fold (Uttanasana): Using blocks under her hands to prevent strain on her lower back.
Downward Dog (Adho Mukha Svanasana): Bending her knees to maintain a neutral spine.
Bridge Pose (Setu Bandhasana): Using a block under her sacrum for support.
Results: Within three months, Sarah reported significant reduction in back pain, improved posture, and increased hamstring flexibility.
Case Study 2: Yoga for Anxiety Management

Profile: John, 30, Graphic Designer

Background: John experiences high levels of anxiety, particularly at work. He sought yoga as a way to manage stress and improve mental health.

Personalized Practice:

Assessment: John's initial practice was unfocused and sporadic. A consistent, calming routine was recommended.
Modifications:
Child's Pose (Balasana): Extended holds with a bolster for deep relaxation.
Seated Forward Bend (Paschimottanasana): Using a strap around his feet and a bolster under his knees for support.
Breathing Exercises (Pranayama): Incorporating Nadi Shodhana (alternate nostril breathing) to reduce anxiety.
Results: John noticed a significant decrease in anxiety levels, better focus, and a sense of calm during stressful situations.
Case Study 3: Yoga for Increased Flexibility
Profile: Emily, 27, Dancer

Background: Emily is a professional dancer with tight hip flexors and hamstrings, looking to improve her flexibility for better performance.

Personalized Practice:

Assessment: Emily's practice focused on deep stretches and dynamic movements.
Modifications:
Pigeon Pose (Eka Pada Rajakapotasana): Using a bolster under her hips to gradually deepen the stretch.
Reclined Hand-to-Big-Toe Pose (Supta Padangusthasana): Using a strap to hold her foot and extending the stretch.

Yin Yoga Poses: Incorporating longer holds to target deep connective tissues.

Results: Over six months, Emily achieved greater flexibility in her hips and hamstrings, enhancing her dance performance.

Case Study 4: Yoga for Weight Loss and Mobility

Profile: Mark, 50, Retired Athlete

Background: Mark struggled with weight gain and reduced mobility post-retirement. He aimed to lose weight and regain mobility through yoga.

Personalized Practice:

Assessment: Focused on building strength, increasing cardiovascular activity, and improving joint mobility.

Modifications:

Warrior II (Virabhadrasana II): Shortening the stance and using a chair for balance.

Sun Salutations (Surya Namaskar): Modified flow with knee-friendly alternatives.

Chair Yoga: Incorporating seated poses to maintain mobility without excessive strain.

Results: Mark lost 15 pounds over eight months and significantly improved his overall mobility and joint health.

Case Study 5: Yoga for Prenatal Health

Profile: Lisa, 32, Pregnant (Second Trimester)

Background: Lisa wanted to maintain her fitness and prepare her body for childbirth while managing common pregnancy-related discomforts.

Personalized Practice:

Assessment: Focused on gentle stretches, relaxation, and strength-building poses safe for pregnancy.

Modifications:

Cat-Cow Pose (Marjaryasana-Bitilasana): To relieve lower back tension.

Goddess Pose (Utkata Konasana): Using a chair for support and stability.

Side-Lying Savasana: For deep relaxation and comfort.

Results: Lisa experienced reduced back pain, better sleep, and a stronger connection to her body and baby.

Conclusion

These case studies illustrate the power of personalized yoga practices tailored to individual needs and conditions. By adapting poses and using modifications, yoga can provide significant physical and mental benefits. The next chapter will explore how yoga can be customized for specific health conditions, offering further insights into the therapeutic potential of this ancient practice.

Readers' Questions and Expert Responses

Q1: How can I apply these case study insights to my own practice?

Response: Start with a self-assessment or consult a yoga instructor to identify your specific needs. Incorporate relevant modifications and poses tailored to your goals. Regularly reassess your practice and progress.

Q2: Can I combine elements from different case studies for a holistic practice?

Response: Absolutely. Combining elements can create a well-rounded practice. For example, integrating relaxation techniques from the anxiety management case study with strength-building from the weight loss case study can address multiple aspects of wellness.

Q3: What if I don't see immediate results?

Response: Patience and consistency are key. Yoga is a gradual process, and changes may take time. Maintain a regular practice, listen to your body, and make adjustments as needed. Celebrate small progressions along the way.
Q4: How do I find a qualified instructor to help personalize my practice?

Response: Look for instructors certified by reputable organizations like Yoga Alliance. Attend classes or workshops to find an instructor whose teaching style resonates with you. Consider private sessions for personalized guidance.
By providing these detailed case studies and addressing common concerns, this chapter aims to inspire and guide readers towards creating a yoga practice that is uniquely tailored to their individual needs.

Chapter 7: Customizing Yoga for Specific Conditions

Yoga has the potential to offer significant benefits for various health conditions when practiced with appropriate modifications. This chapter provides guidance on tailoring yoga practices to address specific medical issues, ensuring safety and effectiveness for practitioners with diverse needs.

Common Health Conditions and Yoga Modifications
1. Back Pain

Challenges: Chronic discomfort, limited mobility.

Modifications:

Cat-Cow Pose (Marjaryasana-Bitilasana): Gentle spinal movement to relieve tension.
Sphinx Pose (Salamba Bhujangasana): Mild backbend to strengthen the lower back.
Child's Pose (Balasana): Use a bolster for support and to alleviate pressure on the spine.
Expert Tips: Focus on core strengthening exercises and maintain gentle, mindful movements to avoid aggravating pain.

2. Arthritis

Challenges: Joint stiffness, pain, reduced range of motion.

Modifications:

Chair Yoga: Perform poses seated or using a chair for support.
Warrior II (Virabhadrasana II): Shorten the stance to reduce
pressure on the knees and hips.
Hand-to-Knee Pose (Janusirsasana): Use a strap around the
foot and a bolster under the knee.
Expert Tips: Emphasize gentle stretching and strengthening to
maintain joint health. Avoid high-impact poses and
movements.

3. Anxiety and Stress

Challenges: High levels of stress, difficulty relaxing, racing
thoughts.

Modifications:

Restorative Poses: Extended holds in poses like Legs-Up-the-
Wall (Viparita Karani) and Supported Reclining Bound Angle
Pose (Supta Baddha Konasana).
Breathing Techniques (Pranayama): Practice deep, rhythmic
breathing exercises such as Nadi Shodhana (alternate nostril
breathing).
Mindfulness Meditation: Integrate short meditation sessions
with the yoga practice.
Expert Tips: Create a calm environment, practice regularly,
and focus on grounding poses that promote relaxation and
mental clarity.

4. High Blood Pressure

Challenges: Need to avoid poses that increase blood pressure.

Modifications:

Forward Bends: Use a chair or blocks to avoid head-down positions.
Gentle Twists: Perform seated or supine twists with minimal spinal rotation.
Supported Poses: Use props for poses like Bridge Pose (Setu Bandhasana) to keep the heart above the head.
Expert Tips: Avoid inversions and high-intensity practices. Focus on slow, controlled movements and calming breathwork.

5. Pregnancy

Challenges: Adjusting to bodily changes, maintaining balance, avoiding poses that compress the belly.

Modifications:

Warrior Poses: Widen the stance and use a chair for support.
Squats (Malasana): Use a block under the hips for support.
Side-Lying Positions: Incorporate side-lying savasana for relaxation.
Expert Tips: Avoid deep backbends, twists, and poses that compress the abdomen. Focus on hip openers, gentle stretches, and breath awareness.

6. Osteoporosis

Challenges: Fragile bones, risk of fractures.

Modifications:

Standing Poses: Use a wall or chair for balance and support.
Avoid Forward Bends: Focus on poses that strengthen the back without forward flexion.

Gentle Backbends: Include supported backbends like Sphinx
Pose (Salamba Bhujangasana) for spinal strengthening.
Expert Tips: Emphasize balance and strength-building poses.
Avoid high-impact or forceful movements.

7. Asthma

Challenges: Breathing difficulties, need for gentle lung
expansion.

Modifications:

Seated Forward Bend (Paschimottanasana): Use a strap
around the feet and a bolster under the knees.
Supported Bridge Pose (Setu Bandhasana): Use a block under
the sacrum.
Breathing Exercises (Pranayama): Practice deep, slow
breathing techniques like Ujjayi (victorious breath).
Expert Tips: Focus on poses that open the chest and improve
lung capacity. Avoid intense or rapid breathwork that could
trigger symptoms.

Personalized Yoga Routines for Specific Conditions
Case Study: Custom Yoga Routine for Back Pain

Profile: Rachel, 35, Office Worker

Condition: Chronic lower back pain from prolonged sitting.

Personalized Routine:

Warm-Up: Cat-Cow Pose (Marjaryasana-Bitilasana) for gentle
spinal movement.
Main Poses: Sphinx Pose (Salamba Bhujangasana), Child's
Pose (Balasana) with bolster, Bridge Pose (Setu Bandhasana)
with block support.

Cool-Down: Legs-Up-the-Wall Pose (Viparita Karani) for relaxation.
Breathwork: Deep belly breathing to promote relaxation and pain relief.
Results: Rachel experienced reduced back pain, improved posture, and greater flexibility after three months of consistent practice.

Addressing Readers' Concerns
Q1: How can I determine which modifications are best for my condition?

Response: Start with a professional assessment from a healthcare provider or certified yoga therapist. They can identify your specific needs and recommend appropriate modifications.
Q2: Are there any conditions where yoga is not advisable?

Response: While yoga can benefit many conditions, certain acute injuries, severe osteoporosis, or advanced cardiovascular conditions may require specific medical clearance before starting a practice. Always consult with a healthcare provider before beginning any new exercise regimen.
Q3: How can I integrate these modifications into my existing yoga routine?

Response: Gradually introduce modifications into your practice, starting with poses that directly address your condition. Listen to your body and adjust as needed. Consider attending specialized yoga classes or workshops for additional guidance.
Q4: Can yoga replace medical treatments for specific conditions?

Response: Yoga can complement but not replace medical treatments. It should be used as part of a holistic approach to health, alongside conventional medical care. Always follow your healthcare provider's recommendations.
Q5: How do I know if I'm performing the modifications correctly?

Response: Practice under the guidance of a certified yoga instructor or therapist, especially when starting. Use mirrors or video recordings to check your alignment, and listen to your body's feedback to ensure comfort and safety.
By customizing yoga practices to suit specific conditions, practitioners can safely and effectively incorporate yoga into their wellness routines, achieving better health outcomes and improved quality of life. The next chapter will explore the long-term effects of yoga, providing a deeper understanding of its benefits over time.

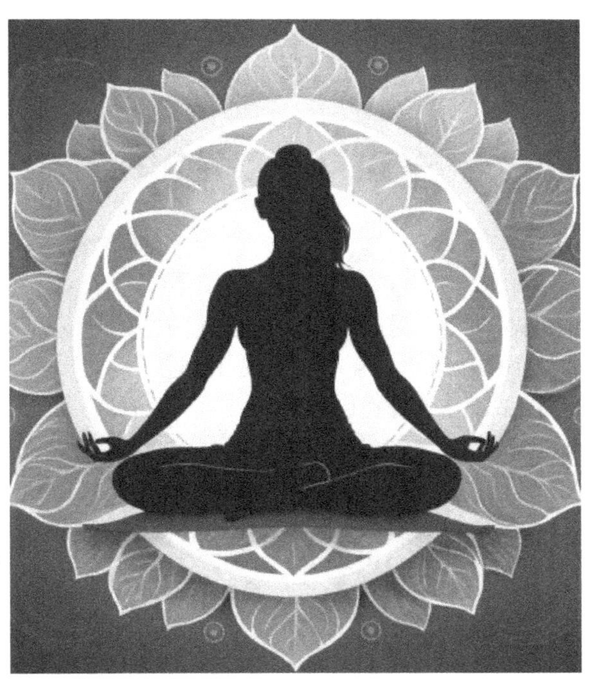

Chapter 8: Tailoring Yoga for Common Health Conditions

Yoga offers tailored approaches to address common health conditions effectively, promoting healing, flexibility, and overall well-being. This chapter explores specific modifications and practices designed to alleviate symptoms and enhance quality of life for individuals managing conditions such as back pain and arthritis.

Yoga for Back Pain Relief
Challenges: Chronic discomfort, limited mobility.

Modifications and Practices:

Cat-Cow Pose (Marjaryasana-Bitilasana): Gentle spinal movement to warm up and alleviate tension.
Bridge Pose (Setu Bandhasana): Using a block under the sacrum to support and strengthen the lower back.
Child's Pose (Balasana): Extended holds with a bolster for deep relaxation and spinal decompression.
Pranayama: Incorporating deep belly breathing (diaphragmatic breathing) to relax and release tension in the back muscles.
Expert Tips: Focus on gradual progression, avoiding deep bends initially, and ensuring proper alignment and support in each pose.

Yoga for Arthritis Management

Challenges: Joint stiffness, pain, reduced range of motion.

Modifications and Practices:

Chair Yoga: Performing seated poses or using a chair for support to reduce pressure on joints.
Gentle Twists: Seated or reclined twists to maintain spinal mobility without strain.
Warrior II (Virabhadrasana II): Shortening the stance and using props for stability to protect knees and hips.
Breathing Exercises: Incorporating slow, controlled breathwork to calm the nervous system and manage pain perception.
Expert Tips: Emphasize gentle stretching and strengthening to improve joint health. Avoid overexertion and listen to your body's limits.

Yoga for Anxiety and Stress Relief
Challenges: High levels of stress, difficulty relaxing, racing thoughts.

Modifications and Practices:

Restorative Poses: Supported versions of forward bends and gentle inversions for relaxation.
Meditation: Guided mindfulness meditation or visualization techniques to calm the mind.
Alternate Nostril Breathing (Nadi Shodhana): Pranayama practice to balance energy and reduce anxiety.
Corpse Pose (Savasana): Extended relaxation to integrate the benefits of the practice.
Expert Tips: Create a tranquil environment, use soft lighting and calming music, and encourage deep, diaphragmatic breathing throughout the practice.

Yoga for High Blood Pressure Management

Challenges: Need to avoid poses that increase blood pressure.

Modifications and Practices:

Seated Poses: Performing seated forward bends and twists to maintain stability and avoid strain.
Supported Inversions: Gentle inversions with props like bolsters under the hips for circulation improvement.
Corpse Pose (Savasana): Using cushions or blankets to elevate the head and chest slightly.
Expert Tips: Focus on poses that promote relaxation and avoid holding the breath. Monitor blood pressure before and after practice.

Yoga for Pregnancy Health
Challenges: Adapting to bodily changes, maintaining balance, avoiding abdominal compression.

Modifications and Practices:

Prenatal Yoga Poses: Gentle stretches and strengthening exercises suitable for each trimester.
Pelvic Floor Exercises: Incorporating Kegel exercises and awareness into the practice.
Modified Twists and Backbends: Using props and modifying depth to accommodate belly size and comfort.
Expert Tips: Avoid deep twists, backbends, and poses that strain the abdomen. Prioritize safety and comfort for both mother and baby.

Yoga for Osteoporosis Management
Challenges: Fragile bones, risk of fractures.

Modifications and Practices:

Gentle Standing Poses: Using props like walls or chairs for balance and stability.
Back Strengthening: Incorporating gentle backbends like Sphinx Pose (Salamba Bhujangasana) with props.
Avoiding High-Impact Poses: Stepping lightly and avoiding jumps or sudden movements.
Expert Tips: Emphasize alignment, avoid forward bends that could strain the spine, and focus on gentle, controlled movements.

Yoga for Asthma Management
Challenges: Breathing difficulties, need for gentle lung expansion.

Modifications and Practices:

Seated and Supine Poses: Performing poses that open the chest without straining the breath.
Supported Poses: Using bolsters or cushions under the back or head for relaxation and ease.
Pranayama Techniques: Practicing slow, rhythmic breathing like Ujjayi Pranayama to improve lung capacity.
Expert Tips: Monitor breath patterns, avoid strenuous poses, and maintain a calm, controlled practice environment.

Conclusion
Tailoring yoga practices to specific health conditions enhances therapeutic benefits and promotes overall well-being. By incorporating these modifications and expert tips, individuals can safely and effectively integrate yoga into their daily routines, managing symptoms and improving quality of life. The next chapter will explore safety measures and injury prevention techniques in yoga, ensuring a safe and sustainable practice for all practitioners.

Chapter 9: Adapting Poses for Individual Needs and Limitations

Yoga is a versatile practice that can be adapted to accommodate various physical abilities, limitations, and individual needs. This chapter explores strategies for modifying yoga poses to ensure accessibility and safety, empowering practitioners to experience the benefits of yoga regardless of their circumstances.

Understanding Individual Needs in Yoga Practice Assessment and Personalization:

Professional Guidance: Consultation with a certified yoga instructor or therapist to assess individual capabilities, limitations, and goals.
Physical Considerations: Factors such as age, flexibility, strength, and any existing health conditions influence pose adaptations.
Strategies for Pose Adaptation
1. Props and Equipment:

Yoga Blocks: Adjusting the height to support stability and alignment in standing poses like Trikonasana (Triangle Pose).
Yoga Straps: Assisting in reaching and maintaining alignment in seated forward bends and binds.

Blankets and Bolsters: Providing comfort and support in restorative poses and relaxation.
2. Modification Principles:

Range of Motion: Adapting the depth and intensity of poses to accommodate joint mobility and flexibility.
Stability and Balance: Using walls, chairs, or props to enhance stability and prevent falls in balancing poses.
Comfort and Support: Incorporating cushions or folded blankets to cushion sensitive areas or support the spine in reclined poses.
3. Pose Variations:

Standing Poses: Adjusting stance width and incorporating chair support for balance in poses like Virabhadrasana (Warrior Pose).
Seated Poses: Using chairs or blocks under the hips to facilitate ease and alignment in poses such as Sukhasana (Easy Pose).
Floor Poses: Utilizing cushions or rolled blankets under knees or back for comfort and alignment in supine or prone positions.
Case Studies: Practical Applications of Pose Adaptation
Case Study 1: Yoga for Seniors

Profile: Margaret, 70, Retired Teacher

Goals: Enhance flexibility, maintain joint health, and reduce stress.

Adaptations:

Chair Yoga: Incorporating seated poses like gentle twists and forward bends to improve mobility and relaxation.
Supported Standing Poses: Using a chair or wall for balance and support in poses such as Tree Pose (Vrksasana).

Breathing Exercises: Practicing seated Pranayama techniques like Dirga Pranayama (Three-Part Breath) for relaxation.
Results: Margaret experienced improved flexibility, reduced joint stiffness, and a greater sense of calm after regular practice.

Case Study 2: Yoga for Individuals with Disabilities

Profile: David, 45, Paraplegic due to spinal injury

Goals: Enhance upper body strength, improve circulation, and promote emotional well-being.

Adaptations:

Wheelchair Yoga: Performing modified poses such as seated twists and gentle arm stretches to enhance mobility and strength.
Breathing Techniques: Practicing Pranayama in a seated position to improve lung capacity and relaxation.
Mindfulness Meditation: Integrating guided meditation practices to support emotional resilience and mental clarity.
Results: David reported increased upper body strength, improved circulation, and enhanced emotional balance through consistent yoga practice.

Addressing Readers' Concerns
Q1: How can I adapt yoga poses if I have limited mobility or flexibility?

Response: Start with gentle modifications and gradually increase depth and intensity as comfort and capability allow. Work with a qualified instructor to tailor poses to your specific needs.
Q2: What if I struggle with balance or stability in certain poses?

Response: Use props such as walls, chairs, or yoga blocks to enhance stability and prevent falls. Focus on maintaining steady breath and mindfulness during practice.
Q3: Can I practice yoga if I have chronic pain or injuries?

Response: Yes, yoga can be adapted to accommodate various injuries and chronic conditions. Consult with a healthcare provider or experienced yoga therapist for personalized guidance.
Q4: How do I know if I'm using props correctly?

Response: Attend classes or workshops led by certified instructors who can demonstrate proper prop usage. Practice under supervision initially to ensure safety and alignment.
Q5: Can yoga help improve flexibility and mobility over time?

Response: Absolutely. Consistent practice with appropriate adaptations can gradually increase flexibility, mobility, and overall well-being. Patience and regularity are key to seeing progress.
Conclusion
Adapting yoga poses for individual needs and limitations enhances accessibility and safety, making yoga a beneficial practice for everyone. By incorporating personalized adaptations and guidance, practitioners can experience the transformative benefits of yoga while honoring their unique physical abilities and circumstances. The next chapter will delve into the long-term effects of yoga on mental and physical health, providing insights into sustained well-being through regular practice.

Chapter 10: Expert Tips on Safe Modifications

Yoga practice is inherently adaptable, allowing practitioners to modify poses to suit individual needs and ensure safety. This chapter focuses on expert tips and guidelines for making modifications that support a sustainable and injury-free yoga practice.

Understanding Safe Modifications
1. Alignment and Awareness:

Importance of proper alignment to prevent strain and injury.
Techniques for cultivating body awareness during practice.
2. Gradual Progression:

Strategies for gradually increasing pose depth and intensity.
Benefits of a progressive approach to avoid overexertion.
3. Prop Utilization:

Overview of commonly used props (blocks, straps, bolsters) and their role in safe modifications.
Specific ways props can enhance stability, alignment, and comfort in poses.
Expert Guidelines for Specific Conditions
1. Back Pain:

Recommended modifications to alleviate spinal discomfort.
Poses to avoid and alternatives for gentle spinal care.
2. Joint Health (Arthritis):

Gentle modifications to protect and support joints.
Importance of maintaining joint mobility and stability.
3. Cardiovascular Health:

Safe practices for individuals with heart conditions.
Poses and techniques to promote cardiovascular health
without strain.
Injury Prevention Strategies
1. Warm-Up and Cool-Down:

Effective warm-up routines to prepare muscles and joints.
Importance of cool-down stretches to promote recovery and
flexibility.
2. Listening to the Body:

Techniques for tuning into physical cues and adjusting
practice accordingly.
Signs of overexertion and when to modify or rest.
Case Studies: Practical Application of Safe Modifications
Case Study 1: Preventing Strain in Yoga Practice

Profile: Sarah, 40, Office Worker

Challenge: Struggling with lower back pain during yoga
practice.

Expert Recommendations:

Warm-Up Routine: Incorporating gentle stretches and
movements to prepare the spine.
Modified Poses: Using props like a bolster in seated forward
bends to avoid excessive spinal flexion.

Alignment Focus: Emphasizing hip alignment and core engagement in standing poses to support the lower back.
Results: Sarah reported reduced discomfort and increased confidence in her yoga practice with consistent application of safe modifications.

Case Study 2: Managing Joint Pain

Profile: Michael, 55, Living with arthritis.

Challenge: Stiffness and discomfort in knees and shoulders during yoga practice.

Expert Recommendations:

Prop Assistance: Utilizing blocks and straps to maintain proper alignment and ease joint strain.
Range-of-Motion Focus: Emphasizing gentle movements to improve flexibility without exacerbating inflammation.
Balancing Strength and Flexibility: Incorporating poses that strengthen surrounding muscles to support joint health.
Results: Michael experienced improved joint mobility and reduced pain with targeted modifications and a focus on gradual progression.

Addressing Readers' Concerns
Q1: How can I modify poses effectively without losing the essence of the practice?

Response: Focus on maintaining breath awareness and mindfulness while making adjustments to suit your body's needs. Seek guidance from a qualified instructor for personalized modifications.
Q2: What are some common mistakes to avoid when modifying poses?

Response: Overstretching, neglecting proper alignment, and pushing beyond comfort are common pitfalls. Start conservatively and increase intensity gradually.

Q3: Can safe modifications still provide a challenging yoga practice?

Response: Absolutely. Safe modifications prioritize alignment and sustainability, allowing for a challenging yet mindful practice that supports long-term progress and well-being.

Q4: How can I integrate safe modifications into a group yoga class?

Response: Communicate openly with the instructor about any physical limitations or concerns. Utilize props and alternative poses suggested during class to maintain safety and alignment.

Q5: Is it necessary to consult with a healthcare provider before making modifications?

Response: It's advisable, especially if you have specific health concerns or conditions. A healthcare provider can offer insights and ensure modifications align with your overall health goals.

Conclusion

Implementing safe modifications in yoga practice enhances accessibility, reduces injury risk, and supports long-term physical and mental well-being. By applying expert tips and guidelines, practitioners can cultivate a sustainable yoga practice that fosters growth, resilience, and overall health. The next chapter will explore the holistic benefits of yoga, highlighting its transformative effects on mental and emotional health.

Chapter 11: Long-term Effects of Yoga

Yoga transcends its immediate benefits by offering profound long-term effects on both mental and physical well-being. This chapter explores the transformative impact of consistent yoga practice over time, supported by scientific research and practitioner insights.

Mental Health Benefits
1. Stress Reduction:

Research Findings: Studies showing yoga's role in lowering cortisol levels and enhancing stress resilience.
Practical Application: Techniques like Yoga Nidra and mindful breathing for stress management.
2. Anxiety and Depression Relief:

Scientific Evidence: Exploration of how yoga influences neurotransmitters and brain chemistry to alleviate symptoms.
Practical Tips: Specific poses and breathing exercises proven effective in clinical settings.
3. Cognitive Function Enhancement:

Neuroplasticity: Yoga's potential to stimulate brain plasticity and improve cognitive function over time.

Mindfulness Practices: Integration of meditation and concentration techniques to enhance mental clarity and focus.
Physical Health Benefits
1. Cardiovascular Health:

Heart Health: Effects of yoga on reducing blood pressure, cholesterol levels, and improving circulation.
Asana Practice: Poses that promote cardiovascular fitness and overall heart health.
2. Strength, Flexibility, and Balance:

Musculoskeletal Benefits: Long-term effects on muscle tone, joint flexibility, and postural alignment.
Age-related Benefits: Yoga's role in maintaining mobility and independence as individuals age.
3. Pain Management:

Chronic Pain: Yoga's effectiveness in managing chronic conditions like back pain, arthritis, and migraines.
Holistic Approaches: Combining asanas, pranayama, and mindfulness for comprehensive pain relief.
Lifestyle and Behavioral Changes
1. Sleep Quality Improvement:

Sleep Disorders: Yoga's impact on regulating sleep patterns and promoting restful sleep.
Relaxation Techniques: Yoga nidra and restorative poses for deep relaxation and sleep induction.
2. Nutrition and Mindful Eating:

Mind-Body Connection: How yoga enhances awareness of nutritional needs and supports mindful eating practices.
Ayurvedic Principles: Integration of Ayurveda to complement yoga practice and dietary choices.
Case Studies: Real-life Transformations
Case Study 1: Weight Management

Profile: Emma, 35, Office Manager

Challenge: Struggling with weight gain and stress-related eating habits.

Yoga Approach: Regular practice of Vinyasa flow combined with mindful eating practices and stress reduction techniques.

Results: Emma achieved sustainable weight loss, improved body awareness, and reduced stress levels through consistent yoga practice.

Case Study 2: Chronic Pain Management

Profile: James, 50, Construction Worker

Challenge: Managing chronic lower back pain and joint stiffness.

Yoga Approach: Incorporation of gentle Hatha yoga poses, therapeutic breathing exercises, and regular meditation.

Results: James experienced reduced pain intensity, improved mobility, and increased overall well-being over time.

Addressing Readers' Concerns
Q1: How long does it take to experience the long-term benefits of yoga?

Response: Benefits vary by individual, but regular practice over several weeks to months often yields noticeable improvements in both physical and mental health.
Q2: Can yoga help with conditions like diabetes and hypertension in the long term?

Response: Yes, yoga's holistic approach supports overall health management and can complement medical treatment for chronic conditions.

Q3: Is there a specific age when it's too late to start yoga for long-term benefits?

Response: Yoga is beneficial at any age, promoting health and well-being throughout life. Modifications can be made to suit individual needs and capabilities.

Q4: How does yoga compare with other forms of exercise in terms of long-term health benefits?

Response: Yoga offers unique benefits such as stress reduction, mindfulness, and flexibility, complementing traditional exercises' cardiovascular and strength training aspects.

Q5: What role does consistency play in experiencing long-term benefits?

Response: Consistent practice is key to reaping the full benefits of yoga. Regularity enhances physical conditioning, mental clarity, and overall quality of life.

Conclusion

Yoga's long-term effects encompass physical resilience, mental clarity, and emotional balance, making it a valuable practice for holistic health maintenance. By exploring the comprehensive benefits supported by scientific research and real-life transformations, this chapter illuminates yoga's potential as a lifelong companion in enhancing well-being. The next chapter will delve into safety measures and injury prevention strategies, ensuring a sustainable and enriching yoga journey for practitioners of all levels.

Chapter 12: Mental Health Benefits of Yoga

Yoga is renowned not only for its physical benefits but also for its profound effects on mental and emotional well-being. This chapter explores in-depth the therapeutic benefits of yoga practices on various aspects of mental health, supported by scientific research and practical insights.

Stress Reduction and Resilience
1. Cortisol Regulation:

Research Findings: Yoga's impact on lowering cortisol levels, the stress hormone, promoting relaxation and resilience.
Practical Application: Techniques such as deep breathing, restorative poses, and meditation for stress relief.
2. Mind-Body Connection:

Psychological Benefits: Enhancing awareness of thoughts, emotions, and physical sensations through mindfulness practices.
Integration in Daily Life: Applying mindfulness off the mat to manage stressors and cultivate emotional balance.
Anxiety and Depression Management

1. Neurochemical Effects:

Serotonin and GABA: Yoga's role in boosting neurotransmitters associated with mood regulation and anxiety reduction.
Clinical Applications: Evidence-based yoga protocols for anxiety disorders and depressive symptoms.
2. Breathwork and Relaxation Techniques:

Pranayama Practices: Breathing exercises to calm the nervous system and promote mental clarity.
Progressive Relaxation: Guided techniques for releasing muscle tension and alleviating anxiety.
Cognitive Function Enhancement
1. Brain Plasticity:

Neuroscientific Insights: How yoga stimulates neural pathways, supporting cognitive flexibility and memory retention.
Focus and Concentration: Techniques like Dharana (focused attention) to improve mental acuity and task performance.
2. Mindfulness Meditation:

Benefits Beyond the Mat: Integration of meditation into yoga practice for sustained attention and emotional regulation.
Neurological Benefits: Studies demonstrating changes in brain structure associated with enhanced mindfulness.
Emotional Regulation and Resilience
1. Emotional Intelligence:

Self-Awareness and Empathy: Yoga practices fostering emotional intelligence and interpersonal relationships.
Compassion Cultivation: Techniques for cultivating self-compassion and empathy towards others.
2. Yoga Nidra and Deep Relaxation:

Psychophysiological Effects: Inducing a state of deep relaxation to reduce emotional reactivity and enhance emotional resilience.
Sleep Enhancement: Benefits of Yoga Nidra for improving sleep quality and managing insomnia.
Case Studies: Real-life Applications
Case Study 1: Anxiety Relief

Profile: Sarah, 30, Marketing Executive

Challenge: Persistent generalized anxiety impacting daily life and work productivity.

Yoga Approach: Regular practice of Hatha yoga combined with mindfulness meditation and breathwork.

Results: Sarah reported reduced anxiety symptoms, increased calmness, and improved focus in her professional and personal life.

Case Study 2: Depression Management

Profile: Mark, 45, Teacher

Challenge: Recurrent depressive episodes affecting mood and motivation.

Yoga Approach: Integration of Vinyasa flow and Yin yoga practices with therapeutic breathing exercises.

Results: Mark experienced enhanced mood stability, decreased depressive symptoms, and a renewed sense of purpose through consistent yoga practice.

Addressing Readers' Concerns

Q1: Can yoga help with severe anxiety disorders or clinical depression?

Response: Yoga, combined with professional guidance and possibly medication, can be an effective adjunct therapy for managing symptoms and promoting emotional well-being.
Q2: How long does it take to notice mental health benefits from yoga practice?

Response: Benefits vary by individual, but regular practice over several weeks to months often yields noticeable improvements in mood, stress levels, and overall mental health.
Q3: Are there specific yoga practices better suited for managing anxiety versus depression?

Response: Practices like gentle Hatha or restorative yoga may be beneficial for anxiety, while energizing Vinyasa or breath-centered practices can aid in managing depressive symptoms. Personal preference and individual response should guide practice choices.
Q4: Can yoga be used as a self-help tool for managing daily stressors?

Response: Absolutely. Mindfulness techniques, breathwork, and simple yoga sequences can empower individuals to cultivate resilience and manage stress effectively on their own.
Q5: What role does consistency play in experiencing mental health benefits from yoga?

Response: Consistent practice fosters neuroplasticity, emotional regulation, and resilience over time, supporting sustainable improvements in mental health and well-being.
Conclusion

Yoga's profound impact on mental health encompasses stress reduction, anxiety and depression management, cognitive enhancement, and emotional resilience. By exploring the scientific foundations and practical applications of yoga practices, this chapter illuminates its potential as a holistic approach to nurturing mental well-being. The next chapter will explore the physical health benefits of yoga, emphasizing its role in enhancing muscular strength, flexibility, and overall vitality.

Chapter 13: Detailed Exploration of Yoga's Impact on Anxiety, Depression, and Stress

Yoga offers a comprehensive approach to managing and alleviating symptoms of anxiety, depression, and stress through a combination of physical postures, breathwork, mindfulness practices, and relaxation techniques. This chapter delves into the specific mechanisms by which yoga influences mental health, supported by scientific research and practical insights.

Understanding Anxiety and Yoga
1. Neurological Effects:

Cortisol Regulation: Yoga's ability to lower cortisol levels, reducing the body's stress response.
GABA Production: Enhancing gamma-aminobutyric acid (GABA), a neurotransmitter that promotes relaxation and reduces anxiety.
2. Breath-Centered Practices:

Pranayama Techniques: Deep breathing exercises to calm the mind, balance emotions, and regulate the autonomic nervous system.
Anxiety-Specific Practices: Techniques like Nadi Shodhana (Alternate Nostril Breathing) for anxiety relief.
Managing Depression with Yoga
1. Mood Regulation:

Serotonin and Endorphin Release: Yoga's impact on increasing serotonin and endorphin levels, promoting mood elevation and emotional balance.
Mindfulness and Acceptance: Practices that cultivate present-moment awareness to alleviate depressive symptoms.
2. Movement and Mindfulness Integration:

Vinyasa Flow and Depression: Dynamic sequences to stimulate circulation, release tension, and uplift mood.
Yin Yoga and Relaxation: Gentle postures to enhance parasympathetic nervous system activity, promoting relaxation and emotional well-being.
Stress Reduction Strategies
1. Relaxation Response:

Yoga Nidra: Guided relaxation techniques to induce deep states of relaxation, reduce stress hormone levels, and enhance overall well-being.
Restorative Yoga: Passive poses supported by props to facilitate physical and mental relaxation, aiding in stress relief.
2. Cognitive Behavioral Approaches:

Yoga and Cognitive Restructuring: Using yoga practice to challenge negative thought patterns and enhance cognitive flexibility.
Positive Affirmations and Mantras: Incorporating affirmations and sacred chants to cultivate positivity and resilience.

Scientific Research and Evidence
1. Clinical Studies: Overview of key studies demonstrating yoga's efficacy in treating anxiety disorders, depression, and stress-related conditions.

Randomized Controlled Trials: Research methodologies and findings supporting yoga as a complementary therapy in mental health care.
Case Studies: Real-life Applications
Case Study 1: Anxiety Management

Profile: Emily, 25, Graduate Student

Challenge: Generalized anxiety affecting academic performance and personal relationships.

Yoga Approach: Incorporation of Hatha yoga postures, daily pranayama practice, and mindfulness meditation.

Results: Emily reported decreased anxiety symptoms, improved focus, and enhanced emotional resilience, enabling better academic achievement and interpersonal connections.

Case Study 2: Depression Relief

Profile: John, 40, IT Professional

Challenge: Persistent depressive symptoms impacting work productivity and quality of life.

Yoga Approach: Weekly attendance in a therapeutic yoga class focusing on gentle poses, deep relaxation techniques, and supportive community.

Results: John experienced reduced feelings of sadness, increased energy levels, and greater job satisfaction through consistent yoga practice and emotional support.

Addressing Readers' Concerns
Q1: Can yoga be used as a primary treatment for severe anxiety or depression?

Response: Yoga is effective as a complementary therapy alongside professional treatment. Consultation with healthcare providers is recommended for comprehensive care.
Q2: How soon can one expect to notice improvements in anxiety or depressive symptoms with yoga practice?

Response: Individual responses vary, but regular practice over several weeks can lead to noticeable reductions in symptoms and improvements in overall well-being.
Q3: What are the best yoga practices for managing acute stress?

Response: Quick, breath-centered practices such as Bhramari Pranayama (Bee Breath) and grounding asanas like Child's Pose can provide immediate relief and calm the nervous system.
Q4: Are there specific yoga styles or approaches better suited for different mental health conditions?

Response: Tailoring yoga practices to individual needs and preferences is key. Gentle, restorative practices may be beneficial for depression, while energizing sequences can aid in managing anxiety.
Q5: How does yoga compare to conventional therapies like medication and psychotherapy in treating mental health disorders?

Response: Yoga complements conventional treatments by addressing both physical and psychological aspects of well-being. Integrative approaches can enhance overall therapeutic outcomes.

Conclusion

Yoga serves as a powerful tool for managing anxiety, depression, and stress, offering holistic approaches that foster emotional resilience and mental clarity. By exploring the specific impacts of yoga practices on mental health and sharing real-life applications, this chapter illuminates yoga's potential as a transformative practice for emotional well-being. The next chapter will examine the physical health benefits of yoga, emphasizing its role in enhancing strength, flexibility, and overall vitality.

Chapter 14: Yoga and Cognitive Function: Beyond Age-Related Memory Loss

Introduction
Overview of the increasing interest in yoga for enhancing cognitive function:

The popularity of yoga has surged globally due to its holistic benefits, including physical, mental, and emotional well-being.
Recent studies suggest yoga's potential in improving cognitive abilities, attracting interest from various age groups, particularly older adults.
Explanation of age-related memory loss and its impact:

Age-related memory loss is a natural part of aging, affecting the ability to recall information and perform daily tasks.
It can lead to frustration, decreased quality of life, and anxiety about developing conditions like dementia.
Yoga's potential beyond mitigating age-related memory decline:

While yoga is known for reducing stress and promoting physical health, its impact on cognitive function is gaining attention.

Yoga may enhance overall cognitive abilities, such as attention, memory, and executive function, beyond merely addressing memory decline.

Section 1: The Science of Yoga and the Brain

Impact of yoga on the brain:

Yoga promotes neuroplasticity, the brain's ability to reorganize and form new neural connections.
It increases gray matter density in brain regions involved in memory, attention, and learning.
Yoga's effect on brain regions related to memory and cognition:

Hippocampus: Critical for forming and retrieving memories; yoga practices like meditation and mindfulness can increase its volume.
Prefrontal Cortex: Associated with decision-making, attention, and executive function; yoga enhances its functioning through stress reduction and improved focus.
Research findings:

Studies show that regular yoga practice can lead to significant improvements in cognitive performance.
Yoga's benefits include better memory recall, enhanced concentration, and improved executive functions.

Section 2: Age-Related Memory Loss: Causes and Challenges

Explanation of age-related memory loss:

Describes normal cognitive aging, characterized by slower information processing and occasional forgetfulness.
Differentiates between normal aging and pathological conditions like Alzheimer's disease.
Causes of age-related memory loss:

Reduced blood flow to the brain.
Decline in neurotransmitters.

Accumulation of free radicals causing oxidative stress.
Common challenges:

Difficulty in learning new information.
Increased time needed to recall names and places.
Misplacing items more frequently.
Distinguishing normal changes from serious conditions:

Normal aging involves mild forgetfulness, while conditions like dementia involve severe memory impairment and confusion.
Section 3: Yoga Practices for Enhancing Cognitive Function
Specific yoga practices:

Asanas (Physical Postures): Improve blood flow to the brain, enhance body awareness, and reduce stress. Examples include:
Sirsasana (Headstand): Increases blood flow to the brain.
Sarvangasana (Shoulder Stand): Enhances thyroid function, which supports cognitive health.
Pranayama (Breathing Exercises): Improve oxygen supply to the brain and reduce anxiety. Examples include:
Nadi Shodhana (Alternate Nostril Breathing): Balances the nervous system.
Kapalabhati (Skull Shining Breath): Energizes the mind.
Meditation and Mindfulness Practices: Enhance focus and reduce cognitive decline. Examples include:
Mindfulness Meditation: Increases attention span and working memory.
Loving-Kindness Meditation: Promotes emotional regulation and reduces stress.
Detailed descriptions and benefits:

Step-by-step guides for each practice.
Explanation of how these practices improve cognitive function.

Tips for integrating these practices into daily routines.
Section 4: Case Studies and Personal Stories
Real-life examples:

Stories of individuals who experienced cognitive improvements through regular yoga practice.
Diverse backgrounds, including older adults, professionals, and students.
Testimonials:

Quotes from practitioners about how yoga improved their memory, focus, and overall cognitive abilities.
Personal insights into how yoga helped them manage age-related memory challenges.
Analysis of benefits:

Examination of how specific yoga practices contributed to their cognitive enhancements.
Discussion of the psychological and emotional benefits experienced.
Section 5: Developing a Yoga Routine for Cognitive Health
Guidelines for creating a personalized routine:

Tailored advice for beginners, intermediate, and advanced practitioners.
Importance of consistency and gradual progression.
Recommendations for different levels:

Beginners: Focus on gentle asanas, simple breathing exercises, and basic meditation practices.
Intermediate: Incorporate more challenging postures, advanced breathing techniques, and longer meditation sessions.
Advanced: Explore complex asanas, pranayama variations, and deep meditation practices.
Safety tips and modifications:

Adjustments for individuals with physical limitations or health conditions.
Emphasis on listening to one's body and avoiding overexertion.
Section 6: Combining Yoga with Other Cognitive-Enhancing Strategies
Complementary strategies:

Nutrition and Diet: Foods that support brain health, such as omega-3 fatty acids, antioxidants, and vitamins.
Mental Exercises: Puzzles, games, and activities that stimulate the brain.
Physical Exercise: Regular aerobic and strength training exercises to boost overall brain function.
Integration for maximum benefit:

Creating a balanced lifestyle that incorporates yoga, proper nutrition, mental exercises, and physical activity.
Tips for maintaining consistency and motivation.

Chapter 15: Physical Health Benefits

Introduction
Overview of Yoga's Physical Health Benefits:
Yoga is widely recognized for its ability to enhance physical health, contributing to a well-rounded approach to wellness. Introduction to the various physical health benefits, ranging from improved flexibility to enhanced cardiovascular health.
Section 1: Enhancing Flexibility and Balance
Importance of Flexibility and Balance:

Flexibility helps prevent injuries, reduces muscle soreness, and improves overall physical performance.
Balance is crucial for preventing falls, especially in older adults, and for enhancing coordination.
Yoga Practices for Flexibility and Balance:

Asanas:
Downward-Facing Dog (Adho Mukha Svanasana): Stretches the hamstrings, calves, and shoulders.
Warrior Pose (Virabhadrasana): Strengthens the legs and improves balance.
Tree Pose (Vrksasana): Enhances balance and concentration.
Tips for Practicing:

Start with gentle stretches and progress gradually.
Use props like yoga blocks and straps for support.
Section 2: Strengthening Muscles and Bones
Building Muscle Strength:

Yoga helps build muscle strength without the strain of lifting heavy weights.
Strengthening muscles supports joint health and enhances overall physical performance.
Supporting Bone Health:

Weight-bearing poses in yoga stimulate bone growth and help prevent osteoporosis.
Key Yoga Poses for Strength:

Plank Pose (Phalakasana): Builds core strength.
Chair Pose (Utkatasana): Strengthens the thighs and glutes.
Bridge Pose (Setu Bandhasana): Strengthens the back and glutes.
Tips for Practicing:

Focus on proper alignment to maximize benefits and prevent injury.
Incorporate a variety of poses to target different muscle groups.
Section 3: Improving Cardiovascular Health
Yoga and Heart Health:

Regular yoga practice can lower blood pressure, reduce cholesterol levels, and improve heart rate variability.
Yoga Practices for Cardiovascular Health:

Vinyasa Flow: A dynamic sequence of poses that increases heart rate and improves circulation.
Breathing Techniques (Pranayama):

Ujjayi Breath: Helps regulate blood pressure and enhance lung capacity.

Nadi Shodhana (Alternate Nostril Breathing): Balances the autonomic nervous system.

Research Findings:

Studies show that yoga can be as effective as aerobic exercise in improving cardiovascular health.

Tips for Practicing:

Start with gentle flows and gradually increase intensity.

Combine yoga with other forms of cardiovascular exercise for optimal benefits.

Section 4: Boosting Immune Function

Yoga's Impact on the Immune System:

Yoga reduces stress hormones that compromise the immune system.

It promotes lymphatic drainage and improves circulation, aiding in the removal of toxins.

Yoga Practices for Immune Health:

Twisting Poses: Aid in detoxification and stimulate the lymphatic system.

Revolved Triangle Pose (Parivrtta Trikonasana)

Seated Spinal Twist (Ardha Matsyendrasana)

Inversions: Improve circulation and support the immune system.

Legs Up the Wall (Viparita Karani)

Shoulder Stand (Sarvangasana)

Tips for Practicing:

Practice restorative poses during periods of illness or fatigue.

Maintain a regular yoga routine to support overall immune function.

Section 5: Enhancing Respiratory Health

Yoga and the Respiratory System:

Yoga improves lung capacity and efficiency.
Breathing exercises enhance respiratory health and reduce symptoms of asthma and other respiratory conditions.
Key Breathing Techniques:

Diaphragmatic Breathing: Strengthens the diaphragm and improves oxygen intake.
Kapalabhati (Skull Shining Breath): Clears the lungs and invigorates the respiratory system.
Yoga Poses for Respiratory Health:

Fish Pose (Matsyasana): Opens the chest and lungs.
Bridge Pose (Setu Bandhasana): Expands the chest and improves breathing.
Tips for Practicing:

Focus on deep, mindful breathing during poses.
Incorporate breathing exercises into your daily routine.
Conclusion
Recap of Key Physical Health Benefits:
Yoga improves flexibility, balance, muscle strength, cardiovascular health, immune function, and respiratory health.

Chapter 16: Cardiovascular Health and Yoga

Introduction
Overview of Cardiovascular Health:
Importance of maintaining a healthy cardiovascular system for overall well-being.
Common cardiovascular issues such as hypertension, heart disease, and stroke.
Introduction to Yoga's Role:
How yoga can play a pivotal role in promoting cardiovascular health.
Summary of the chapter's focus on the relationship between yoga and cardiovascular health.
Section 1: Understanding Cardiovascular Health
The Cardiovascular System:

Components: Heart, blood vessels (arteries, veins, capillaries), and blood.
Functions: Transporting oxygen, nutrients, hormones, and removing waste products.
Common Cardiovascular Problems:

Hypertension: High blood pressure, its causes, and effects.
Heart Disease: Types, such as coronary artery disease, and their impact.
Stroke: Causes, symptoms, and prevention.
Risk Factors:

Lifestyle choices (diet, exercise, smoking).
Genetic predispositions.
Stress and its effects on heart health.
Section 2: The Science Behind Yoga and Cardiovascular Health
How Yoga Benefits the Heart:

Stress Reduction: Yoga lowers cortisol levels, reducing stress and its negative impact on the heart.
Improved Circulation: Yoga enhances blood flow and reduces arterial stiffness.
Lower Blood Pressure: Regular practice can reduce systolic and diastolic blood pressure.
Heart Rate Variability: Yoga improves heart rate variability, indicating better autonomic function.
Research Findings:

Studies showing yoga's effectiveness in reducing cardiovascular risk factors.
Comparative studies between yoga and other forms of exercise on heart health.
Section 3: Yoga Practices for Cardiovascular Health
Asanas (Postures):

Mountain Pose (Tadasana): Improves posture and reduces stress.
Warrior II (Virabhadrasana II): Strengthens the heart and lungs.

Bridge Pose (Setu Bandhasana): Opens the chest and improves circulation.
Legs Up the Wall (Viparita Karani): Calms the mind and reduces blood pressure.
Pranayama (Breathing Exercises):

Diaphragmatic Breathing: Promotes relaxation and lowers heart rate.
Ujjayi Breath (Ocean Breath): Enhances oxygen intake and reduces stress.
Nadi Shodhana (Alternate Nostril Breathing): Balances the autonomic nervous system and lowers blood pressure.
Meditation and Relaxation Techniques:

Mindfulness Meditation: Reduces stress and improves cardiovascular function.
Guided Relaxation (Yoga Nidra): Lowers heart rate and blood pressure.
Tips for Practicing:

Importance of consistency and mindfulness in practice.
Modifications for individuals with cardiovascular issues.
Combining yoga with other heart-healthy practices (e.g., diet, regular check-ups).
Section 4: Case Studies and Personal Stories
Real-Life Examples:

Individuals who have improved their cardiovascular health through yoga.
Stories from people of different ages and backgrounds.
Testimonials:

Personal insights on how yoga helped manage hypertension, reduce stress, and improve overall heart health.
Analysis of specific yoga practices and their impact.
Section 5: Developing a Yoga Routine for Heart Health

Guidelines for Creating a Personalized Routine:

Assessing individual needs and health conditions.
Balancing different types of yoga practices (asanas, pranayama, meditation).
Sample Routines:

Beginner Routine: Gentle poses, basic breathing exercises, and short meditation sessions.
Intermediate Routine: More challenging postures, advanced breathing techniques, and longer meditation.
Advanced Routine: Complex asanas, pranayama variations, and deep meditation practices.
Safety Considerations:

Listening to the body and avoiding overexertion.
Consulting healthcare providers before starting a new yoga regimen, especially for individuals with existing cardiovascular conditions.
Conclusion
Recap of Key Points:
Summary of yoga's benefits for cardiovascular health.
Encouragement to incorporate yoga into daily life for long-term heart health.

Testimonials
Testimonial 1: "Transforming My Life and Heart Health"
Name: Sarah T.
Age: 54

"After being diagnosed with hypertension at 50, I knew I
needed to make some serious changes in my life. I was
introduced to yoga through a friend and started with a
beginner's class. Initially, I was skeptical about its impact on
my heart health, but within a few months, I noticed significant
improvements. My blood pressure began to stabilize, and I felt
more relaxed and in control. The combination of deep
breathing exercises and gentle poses became a daily routine
for me. Today, four years later, my blood pressure is within a
healthy range, and I feel more energetic and optimistic about
life. Yoga has truly transformed my life and heart health."

Testimonial 2: "Finding Balance and Peace"
Name: David M.
Age: 67

"As I entered my 60s, I started experiencing various health issues, including high blood pressure and high cholesterol. My doctor recommended medication, but I wanted to explore natural ways to manage my health. I started practicing yoga after reading about its benefits. The meditation and breathing exercises, especially alternate nostril breathing, helped me manage stress better. Over time, I incorporated more physical poses into my routine. Not only did my blood pressure drop, but my cholesterol levels also improved. Yoga has helped me find balance and peace, and I believe it's been a key factor in maintaining my heart health."

Testimonial 3: "Rejuvenated and Stronger Heart"
Name: Emily R.
Age: 45

"Working in a high-stress environment had taken a toll on my heart. I often felt anxious and had trouble sleeping, which led to elevated blood pressure. A friend suggested yoga, and I decided to give it a try. Starting with basic asanas and pranayama, I gradually noticed changes. My anxiety levels decreased, I slept better, and my heart felt stronger. Regular practice of poses like the Bridge Pose and Legs Up the Wall, combined with mindful breathing, made a significant difference. Now, yoga is an essential part of my life. My heart health has improved, and I feel rejuvenated every day."

Testimonial 4: "A New Beginning with Yoga"
Name: Mark S.
Age: 60

"After a minor heart attack, my cardiologist recommended lifestyle changes, including stress management. I turned to yoga as a holistic approach to recovery. Starting with gentle yoga and breathing exercises, I slowly regained my strength and confidence. Poses like Warrior II and mindful meditation sessions helped me stay focused and calm. Over the past two years, my heart health has significantly improved. Regular yoga practice has not only strengthened my heart but also improved my overall well-being. Yoga gave me a new beginning and a healthier heart."

Testimonial 5: "Healing Through Yoga"
Name: Priya K.
Age: 50

"I have always been an active person, but stress from work and family responsibilities led to high blood pressure and heart palpitations. I tried various methods to manage stress, but nothing seemed to work until I discovered yoga. Incorporating yoga into my daily routine has been a game-changer. Poses like the Mountain Pose and Child's Pose, combined with Ujjayi breathing, have been incredibly soothing. My blood pressure is now under control, and I no longer experience palpitations. Yoga has been my healing journey, giving me a healthier heart and a calmer mind."

These testimonials showcase the diverse experiences of individuals who have benefitted from yoga in improving their cardiovascular health. Their stories highlight the transformative power of yoga in managing stress, lowering blood pressure, and enhancing overall heart health.

Sample Yoga Routines for Cardiovascular Health
Beginner Routine
Duration: 20-30 minutes

Frequency: 3-4 times a week

Equipment: Yoga mat, comfortable clothing, optional yoga block

Warm-Up (5 minutes):

Mountain Pose (Tadasana):

Stand with feet together, arms at sides.
Distribute weight evenly across both feet.
Lengthen through the spine, reaching the crown of the head upward.
Hold for 1-2 minutes, focusing on deep, even breaths.
Cat-Cow Stretch (Marjaryasana-Bitilasana):

Start on hands and knees, wrists under shoulders, knees under hips.
Inhale, arch the back (Cow Pose), lifting the tailbone and chest.
Exhale, round the back (Cat Pose), tucking the chin and tailbone.
Repeat for 5-10 breaths.
Main Practice (15-20 minutes):

Downward-Facing Dog (Adho Mukha Svanasana):

From hands and knees, lift hips up and back.
Form an inverted V-shape with the body.
Press hands into the mat, lengthen the spine, and engage the legs.
Hold for 5-7 breaths.
Warrior II (Virabhadrasana II):

Stand with feet wide apart, turn right foot out and left foot slightly in.
Bend right knee, keeping it above the ankle.
Extend arms out to the sides, gaze over right hand.
Hold for 5-7 breaths, then switch sides.
Bridge Pose (Setu Bandhasana):

Lie on back, bend knees, feet hip-width apart, and close to the hips.
Press feet and arms into the mat, lift hips toward the ceiling.
Interlace fingers under the back and press arms down.
Hold for 5-7 breaths.
Legs Up the Wall (Viparita Karani):

Sit with one side against the wall, then swing legs up as you lie back.
Adjust so hips are close to the wall, legs extended upward.
Relax arms at sides, close eyes, and breathe deeply.

Hold for 5-10 minutes.
Cool Down (5 minutes):

Corpse Pose (Savasana):
Lie flat on your back, arms at sides, palms facing up.
Let feet fall open, close eyes, and focus on relaxing each part
of the body.
Stay in this pose for 5-10 minutes, breathing naturally.
Intermediate Routine
Duration: 30-45 minutes

Frequency: 4-5 times a week

Warm-Up (5 minutes):

Mountain Pose (Tadasana):

Follow the same instructions as the beginner routine.
Hold for 1-2 minutes.
Sun Salutation A (Surya Namaskar A):

Stand at the top of the mat, inhale and raise arms overhead.
Exhale, fold forward, placing hands on the mat.
Inhale, lift halfway up, lengthening the spine.
Exhale, step back to plank, lower down to Chaturanga.
Inhale, lift into Upward-Facing Dog (Urdhva Mukha
Svanasana).
Exhale, transition to Downward-Facing Dog (Adho Mukha
Svanasana).
Repeat for 3-5 cycles.
Main Practice (20-30 minutes):

Warrior I (Virabhadrasana I):

Stand with feet wide apart, turn right foot out, and left foot in.
Bend right knee, raise arms overhead, palms facing each other.

Square hips to the front, hold for 5-7 breaths, then switch sides.
Triangle Pose (Trikonasana):

Stand with feet wide apart, turn right foot out, left foot slightly in.
Extend right arm forward, then lower it to the shin or a block, left arm up.
Gaze up at the left hand, hold for 5-7 breaths, then switch sides.
Camel Pose (Ustrasana):

Kneel with knees hip-width apart, hands on lower back.
Inhale, lift chest, arch back, and reach for the heels.
Press hips forward, lengthen the spine, hold for 5-7 breaths.
Seated Forward Bend (Paschimottanasana):

Sit with legs extended, spine straight.
Inhale, lengthen the spine, exhale, fold forward reaching for feet or shins.
Hold for 5-10 breaths.
Cool Down (5-10 minutes):

Reclining Bound Angle Pose (Supta Baddha Konasana):

Lie on your back, bring soles of the feet together, let knees fall open.
Place hands on the belly or extend them out to the sides.
Close eyes, relax for 5-10 minutes.
Corpse Pose (Savasana):

Follow the same instructions as the beginner routine.
Stay in this pose for 5-10 minutes, focusing on deep relaxation.
Advanced Routine
Duration: 45-60 minutes

Frequency: 5-6 times a week

Warm-Up (5-10 minutes):

Mountain Pose (Tadasana):

Follow the same instructions as the beginner routine.
Hold for 1-2 minutes.
Sun Salutation B (Surya Namaskar B):

Stand at the top of the mat, inhale, bend knees, and come into
Chair Pose (Utkatasana).
Exhale, fold forward, placing hands on the mat.
Inhale, lift halfway up, lengthening the spine.
Exhale, step back to plank, lower down to Chaturanga.
Inhale, lift into Upward-Facing Dog (Urdhva Mukha
Svanasana).
Exhale, transition to Downward-Facing Dog (Adho Mukha
Svanasana).
Inhale, step right foot forward, come into Warrior I
(Virabhadrasana I).
Exhale, step back to plank, repeat sequence on the left side.
Repeat for 3-5 cycles.
Main Practice (30-40 minutes):

Extended Side Angle Pose (Utthita Parsvakonasana):

From Warrior II, lower right hand to the floor or a block
outside the right foot, left arm overhead.
Gaze up at the left hand, hold for 5-7 breaths, then switch
sides.
Half Moon Pose (Ardha Chandrasana):

From Warrior II, shift weight onto the right foot, lift the left
leg parallel to the floor.

Extend the right hand to the floor or a block, left arm up, gaze up.
Hold for 5-7 breaths, then switch sides.
Crow Pose (Bakasana):

Squat down, place hands on the mat, shoulder-width apart.
Lift hips, place knees on the upper arms, and shift weight forward.
Lift feet off the mat, balancing on the hands, hold for 5-7 breaths.
Headstand (Sirsasana):

Kneel, interlace fingers, place forearms on the mat, creating a triangle.
Place the crown of the head in the hands, lift hips, walk feet closer, and lift legs up.
Balance for 10-15 breaths, then lower down gently.
Cool Down (5-10 minutes):

Pigeon Pose (Eka Pada Rajakapotasana):

From Downward-Facing Dog, bring the right knee forward to the right wrist, extend the left leg back.
Square hips to the front, fold forward, and relax.
Hold for 5-10 breaths, then switch sides.
Reclining Twist (Supta Matsyendrasana):

Lie on your back, hug knees to chest, drop them to the right, arms out to the sides.
Gaze to the left, hold for 5-10 breaths, then switch sides.
Corpse Pose (Savasana):

Follow the same instructions as the beginner routine.
Stay in this pose for 5-10 minutes, focusing on deep relaxation.

These routines provide a structured approach to incorporating yoga into your lifestyle for cardiovascular health, tailored to different levels of experience. Remember to listen to your body, avoid overexertion, and consult with a healthcare provider if you have any medical conditions.

Meditation and Relaxation Techniques for Cardiovascular Health
Meditation Techniques
1. Mindfulness Meditation

Purpose: Reduce stress, improve focus, and enhance emotional regulation.
Instructions:
Find a Comfortable Position: Sit or lie down in a comfortable position. Close your eyes.
Focus on Your Breath: Bring your attention to your breath. Notice the sensation of air entering and leaving your nostrils or the rise and fall of your chest.
Observe Thoughts and Emotions: As thoughts or emotions arise, acknowledge them without judgment and gently bring your focus back to your breath.
Duration: Start with 5 minutes and gradually increase to 20-30 minutes.

2. Loving-Kindness Meditation (Metta)

Purpose: Cultivate compassion and positive emotions, reduce anxiety and stress.
Instructions:
Find a Comfortable Position: Sit or lie down comfortably. Close your eyes.
Generate Loving-Kindness: Begin by silently repeating phrases such as "May I be happy, may I be healthy, may I be safe, may I live with ease."
Expand to Others: Gradually extend these wishes to loved ones, acquaintances, and even those with whom you have difficulties.
Duration: Practice for 10-15 minutes, focusing on the feeling of love and kindness.
3. Body Scan Meditation

Purpose: Increase body awareness, reduce stress, and promote relaxation.
Instructions:
Find a Comfortable Position: Lie down on your back with arms at your sides and legs extended.
Focus on Each Body Part: Starting from your toes, bring your attention to each part of your body. Notice any sensations, tension, or relaxation.
Release Tension: As you focus on each part, consciously release any tension. Move slowly up through your body to the top of your head.
Duration: Spend about 20-30 seconds on each body part, taking 10-20 minutes in total.
4. Guided Visualization

Purpose: Reduce stress and anxiety, promote relaxation, and enhance well-being.
Instructions:

Find a Comfortable Position: Sit or lie down comfortably.
Close your eyes.
Create a Peaceful Image: Imagine a serene place, such as a
beach, forest, or meadow. Use all your senses to make the
image vivid.
Explore the Scene: Mentally explore the scene, noticing the
sights, sounds, smells, and sensations.
Duration: Spend 10-20 minutes in your visualization, enjoying
the peacefulness and relaxation it brings.
Relaxation Techniques
1. Progressive Muscle Relaxation (PMR)

Purpose: Reduce physical tension and stress, promote
relaxation.
Instructions:
Find a Comfortable Position: Lie down or sit comfortably.
Close your eyes.
Tense and Relax Muscle Groups: Starting from your toes,
tense each muscle group for 5-10 seconds, then release and
relax for 15-20 seconds. Move progressively through your
body up to your head.
Focus on Relaxation: As you release each muscle group, focus
on the sensation of relaxation and let go of any remaining
tension.
Duration: Complete the entire process in 10-15 minutes.
2. Deep Breathing (Diaphragmatic Breathing)

Purpose: Reduce stress, lower blood pressure, and promote
relaxation.
Instructions:
Find a Comfortable Position: Sit or lie down comfortably.
Place one hand on your chest and the other on your abdomen.
Inhale Deeply: Breathe in slowly through your nose, allowing
your abdomen to rise (not your chest).
Exhale Slowly: Exhale through your mouth, feeling your
abdomen fall.

Repeat: Continue for 5-10 minutes, focusing on deep, steady breaths.
3. Yoga Nidra (Guided Relaxation)

Purpose: Induce deep relaxation, reduce stress, and improve sleep quality.
Instructions:
Find a Comfortable Position: Lie down on your back in Savasana (Corpse Pose) with arms at sides and legs extended.
Set an Intention: Mentally repeat a positive intention or resolve for your practice.
Guided Relaxation: Follow a guided Yoga Nidra script or recording that takes you through body awareness, breath awareness, and visualization.
Duration: Practice for 20-45 minutes, remaining still and focusing on the guidance.
4. Breath Counting

Purpose: Improve focus, reduce stress, and promote relaxation.
Instructions:
Find a Comfortable Position: Sit or lie down comfortably. Close your eyes.
Focus on Breathing: Take a few deep breaths to settle in.
Count Each Breath: On each exhale, count silently (one to ten). When you reach ten, start over at one.
Return to Counting: If your mind wanders, gently bring your focus back to counting.
Duration: Practice for 10-15 minutes, maintaining a steady and relaxed breath.
Implementing the Techniques
Beginner Meditation Routine:

Mindfulness Meditation: 5 minutes
Deep Breathing: 5 minutes
Total Time: 10 minutes

Intermediate Meditation Routine:

Loving-Kindness Meditation: 10 minutes
Progressive Muscle Relaxation: 10 minutes
Total Time: 20 minutes
Advanced Meditation Routine:

Guided Visualization: 10 minutes
Yoga Nidra: 30 minutes
Total Time: 40 minutes
These meditation and relaxation techniques can be tailored to individual needs and schedules, providing a flexible approach to enhancing cardiovascular health and overall well-being.

Chapter 17: Yoga for Strength, Flexibility, and Balance Over the Long Term

Introduction
Maintaining physical strength, flexibility, and balance is crucial for overall health and well-being, especially as we age. Yoga is an effective and holistic practice that enhances these attributes through a combination of physical postures (asanas), breathing techniques (pranayama), and mindfulness. This guide provides a comprehensive explanation of how yoga supports long-term physical health, detailing the benefits and offering practical advice on incorporating these practices into your daily routine.

Understanding Strength, Flexibility, and Balance
Importance of Physical Strength:

Muscle Health: Strong muscles are essential for performing everyday tasks, maintaining posture, and preventing injuries. Yoga helps build and maintain muscle strength through various poses that require muscle engagement and endurance. Aging and Muscle Mass: As we age, muscle mass tends to decrease, a condition known as sarcopenia. Regular yoga practice can help counteract this by promoting muscle retention and growth.
Benefits of Flexibility:

Joint Health: Flexibility exercises improve joint mobility, reduce stiffness, and decrease the risk of joint-related issues. Yoga stretches target different muscle groups and connective tissues, enhancing overall mobility.
Mobility: Improved flexibility allows for more efficient and graceful movements, making daily activities easier and reducing the risk of injury.
The Role of Balance:

Fall Prevention: Good balance is critical for preventing falls, especially in older adults. Yoga poses that challenge and improve balance can significantly reduce the risk of falls. Neuromuscular Coordination: Balance exercises in yoga enhance neuromuscular coordination, leading to better control over body movements and increased stability.
The Science Behind Yoga's Benefits
Yoga and Muscle Strength:

Isometric Contractions: Many yoga poses involve holding positions for extended periods, engaging muscles through isometric contractions. This builds strength and endurance.

Functional Movements: Yoga emphasizes functional movements that mimic everyday activities, helping to build strength in practical and applicable ways.
Yoga and Flexibility:

Stretch Reflex: Yoga stretches are performed slowly and mindfully, allowing muscles to relax and lengthen without triggering the stretch reflex, which can cause muscle contraction and limit flexibility.
Fascia Health: Regular yoga practice helps maintain the health and elasticity of fascia, the connective tissue that surrounds muscles and organs, contributing to overall flexibility.
Yoga and Balance:

Proprioception: Yoga enhances proprioception, the body's ability to sense its position and movement in space. Improved proprioception leads to better balance and coordination.
Core Stability: Many yoga poses strengthen the core muscles, which are essential for maintaining balance and stability.
Research Findings:

Studies have shown that regular yoga practice can improve muscle strength, flexibility, and balance. For example, research published in the "Journal of Strength and Conditioning Research" found that participants who practiced yoga for 12 weeks showed significant improvements in these areas compared to a control group.
Yoga Practices for Strength, Flexibility, and Balance
Asanas (Postures) for Strength:

Plank Pose (Phalakasana):

How to Do It: Start in a push-up position with arms straight and hands under shoulders. Engage the core, keeping the body in a straight line from head to heels.
Benefits: Builds core, shoulder, and arm strength.

Duration: Hold for 30 seconds to 1 minute.
Warrior III (Virabhadrasana III):

How to Do It: Stand on one leg, extend the other leg back, and lower the torso forward, arms reaching ahead.
Benefits: Strengthens legs, core, and improves balance.
Duration: Hold each side for 30 seconds to 1 minute.
Chair Pose (Utkatasana):

How to Do It: Stand with feet together, bend knees, and lower hips as if sitting back into a chair. Raise arms overhead.
Benefits: Strengthens thighs, calves, and back.
Duration: Hold for 1 minute.
Asanas (Postures) for Flexibility:

Downward-Facing Dog (Adho Mukha Svanasana):

How to Do It: From hands and knees, lift hips up and back, forming an inverted V-shape.
Benefits: Stretches hamstrings, calves, and shoulders.
Duration: Hold for 1-2 minutes.
Seated Forward Bend (Paschimottanasana):

How to Do It: Sit with legs extended, spine straight. Inhale, lengthen the spine, exhale, fold forward reaching for feet or shins.
Benefits: Stretches the spine, hamstrings, and calves.
Duration: Hold for 1-2 minutes.
Cobra Pose (Bhujangasana):

How to Do It: Lie face down, hands under shoulders. Inhale, lift chest and head, extending the spine.
Benefits: Stretches the chest, shoulders, and abdomen.
Duration: Hold for 30 seconds to 1 minute.
Asanas (Postures) for Balance:

Tree Pose (Vrksasana):

How to Do It: Stand on one leg, place the sole of the other foot against the inner thigh or calf, and balance. Raise arms overhead.
Benefits: Enhances balance and strengthens legs.
Duration: Hold each side for 30 seconds to 1 minute.
Eagle Pose (Garudasana):

How to Do It: Stand on one leg, wrap the other leg around the standing leg. Cross arms at elbows, bringing palms together.
Benefits: Improves balance, focus, and stretches shoulders and hips.
Duration: Hold each side for 30 seconds to 1 minute.
Half Moon Pose (Ardha Chandrasana):

How to Do It: From Warrior II, shift weight onto the front leg, lift the back leg parallel to the floor, and extend the top arm up.
Benefits: Enhances balance and strengthens legs and core.
Duration: Hold each side for 30 seconds to 1 minute.
Combined Practices for Overall Benefits:

Sun Salutations (Surya Namaskar): A sequence that combines strength, flexibility, and balance.
How to Do It: Perform a series of poses in a flowing sequence, including Mountain Pose, Forward Bend, Plank, Upward-Facing Dog, and Downward-Facing Dog.
Benefits: Improves overall physical health.
Repetitions: Perform 5-10 rounds.
Pranayama (Breathing Exercises):

Ujjayi Breath (Ocean Breath):

How to Do It: Inhale and exhale through the nose, slightly constricting the throat to create a soft hissing sound.

Benefits: Improves focus and endurance during poses.
Alternate Nostril Breathing (Nadi Shodhana):

How to Do It: Close the right nostril with the thumb, inhale through the left nostril. Close the left nostril with the ring finger, exhale through the right nostril. Inhale through the right nostril, then switch and exhale through the left.
Benefits: Balances energy and enhances concentration.
Long-Term Practice and Progression
Creating a Sustainable Yoga Routine:

Consistency: Regular practice is key to reaping long-term benefits. Aim for at least 3-4 sessions per week.
Progression: Gradually increase the intensity and duration of your practice as you build strength, flexibility, and balance.
Adapting Practice Over Time:

Listening to Your Body: Modify poses as needed to accommodate physical changes and prevent injury.
Using Props: Utilize yoga blocks, straps, and blankets to support poses and ensure proper alignment.
Combining Yoga with Other Activities:

Complementary Exercises: Incorporate strength training, cardio, and flexibility exercises alongside yoga for a well-rounded fitness routine.
Rest and Recovery: Ensure adequate rest to prevent injury and support muscle recovery.
Tracking Progress:

Setting Goals: Establish short-term and long-term goals for strength, flexibility, and balance.
Self-Assessment: Regularly assess physical capabilities and adjust routines accordingly.
Case Studies and Personal Stories
Real-Life Examples:

Stories from individuals who have maintained their physical health through long-term yoga practice.
Diverse backgrounds showcasing yoga's universal benefits.
Testimonials:

Personal insights on how yoga has enhanced strength, flexibility, and balance.
Specific examples of yoga practices and their impact.
Conclusion
Recap of Key Points:

Summary of yoga's benefits for long-term physical health. Encouragement to incorporate yoga into daily life for sustained strength, flexibility, and balance.

Testimonials
Testimonial 1: Reclaiming Strength and Mobility
Name: Sarah Thompson
Age: 68
Occupation: Retired Teacher

"Before I started practicing yoga, I struggled with joint pain and stiffness that made everyday tasks difficult. My daughter suggested yoga, and it has been life-changing. Through regular practice, I've regained my strength and flexibility. I can now move with ease and confidence. Yoga has given me a new lease on life, allowing me to enjoy my retirement without physical limitations. I highly recommend it to anyone looking to improve their physical health over the long term."

Testimonial 2: Building Balance and Preventing Falls
Name: Robert Jenkins

Age: 74
Occupation: Retired Engineer

"As I got older, I noticed my balance wasn't as good as it used to be, and I started to worry about falling. I joined a yoga class specifically designed for seniors, and the results have been remarkable. Not only has my balance improved significantly, but I also feel stronger and more stable. The gentle yet effective poses have helped me build core strength and improve my coordination. I haven't had a fall since starting yoga, and I feel more secure in my daily activities."

Testimonial 3: A Journey to Flexibility and Pain Relief
Name: Maria Lopez
Age: 55
Occupation: Office Manager

"I've always had a sedentary job, which led to chronic back pain and stiffness. A friend recommended yoga, and I was skeptical at first. However, after a few months of consistent practice, I noticed a huge difference. My flexibility has improved, and my back pain has significantly decreased. The stretches and poses have loosened up my muscles and joints, making me feel more agile and comfortable. Yoga has become an essential part of my routine, and I can't imagine my life without it."

Testimonial 4: Enhancing Overall Well-being and Fitness
Name: David Williams
Age: 60
Occupation: Entrepreneur

"I started yoga to complement my other fitness activities, and it has exceeded my expectations. Not only has it helped with my strength and flexibility, but it has also improved my mental clarity and stress levels. Yoga offers a perfect balance of physical challenge and relaxation, making it an ideal practice for overall well-being. I feel more balanced, both physically and mentally, and it has positively impacted every aspect of my life. I encourage everyone to give yoga a try, no matter their age or fitness level."

Testimonial 5: Overcoming Physical Limitations and Gaining Confidence
Name: Linda Davis
Age: 62
Occupation: Nurse

"After a knee injury, I was worried about my mobility and ability to stay active. My physical therapist recommended yoga as part of my recovery process. I was amazed at how gentle yet effective it was. Yoga helped me rebuild strength in my legs and improve my flexibility without putting too much strain on my knee. I've regained my confidence in my physical abilities and can now enjoy activities I thought I'd never do again. Yoga has been an empowering journey for me, helping me overcome my physical limitations and live a more active life."

Testimonial 6: Transforming Health with Consistent Practice
Name: John Roberts
Age: 58
Occupation: Financial Analyst

"Consistency is key, and yoga has taught me that. I started yoga to address my back pain and stress, but it has given me so much more. With regular practice, I've seen improvements in my strength, flexibility, and overall health. I feel more balanced and in tune with my body. The breathing exercises have also helped me manage stress better. Yoga has transformed my health, and I highly recommend it to anyone looking to improve their physical and mental well-being over the long term."

Testimonial 7: Rediscovering Physical Freedom
Name: Barbara Nguyen
Age: 65
Occupation: Retired Nurse

"Yoga has been a revelation for me. I used to struggle with stiffness and limited mobility, which affected my quality of life. Since starting yoga, I've rediscovered a sense of physical freedom. The poses and stretches have improved my flexibility, and I feel more agile and capable. Yoga has also helped me build strength, especially in my core and legs, making everyday activities much easier. It's never too late to start, and I encourage anyone looking to improve their physical health to give yoga a try."

These testimonials illustrate the transformative impact yoga can have on individuals' strength, flexibility, and balance, highlighting the practice's long-term benefits for physical health and overall well-being.

Step-by-Step Yoga Poses
1. Plank Pose (Phalakasana)
Purpose: Strengthens the core, shoulders, and arms.

Step-by-Step Instructions:

Starting Position: Begin on your hands and knees. Align your
wrists directly under your shoulders and your knees under
your hips.
Extend Your Legs: Step your feet back one at a time,
straightening your legs and coming onto the balls of your feet.
Your body should form a straight line from your head to your
heels.
Engage the Core: Tighten your abdominal muscles to avoid
sagging in your lower back.
Align Your Body: Keep your neck in a neutral position, gazing
slightly forward.
Hold the Pose: Maintain this position, keeping your body
straight and strong. Hold for 30 seconds to 1 minute,
breathing steadily.
Modifications:

Easier: Lower your knees to the floor while keeping a straight line from head to knees.
Harder: Lift one leg off the floor and hold.
2. Downward-Facing Dog (Adho Mukha Svanasana)
Purpose: Stretches the hamstrings, calves, and shoulders; strengthens the arms and legs.

Step-by-Step Instructions:

Starting Position: Begin on your hands and knees. Align your wrists under your shoulders and your knees under your hips.
Lift Your Hips: Tuck your toes under and lift your hips towards the ceiling, straightening your legs and forming an inverted V-shape.
Adjust Your Hands and Feet: Spread your fingers wide and press firmly into the mat. Your hands should be shoulder-width apart, and your feet hip-width apart.
Engage Your Legs: Press your heels toward the floor and gently straighten your legs without locking your knees.
Align Your Spine: Lengthen your spine by pushing your hips up and back. Relax your head and neck.
Hold the Pose: Stay here for 1-2 minutes, breathing deeply.
Modifications:

Easier: Bend your knees slightly if your hamstrings are tight.
Harder: Lift one leg towards the ceiling for a Three-Legged Downward Dog.
3. Warrior III (Virabhadrasana III)
Purpose: Strengthens the legs, core, and improves balance.

Step-by-Step Instructions:

Starting Position: Stand tall with your feet together and arms at your sides.
Shift Your Weight: Transfer your weight onto your left foot.

Lift Your Right Leg: Extend your right leg straight back while simultaneously leaning your torso forward.

Balance and Align: Your body should form a straight line from your head to your raised foot. Extend your arms forward or bring them to your chest in prayer position.

Engage Your Core: Keep your core muscles tight to maintain balance.

Hold the Pose: Stay here for 30 seconds to 1 minute, then slowly return to standing and repeat on the other side.

Modifications:

Easier: Place your hands on a chair or wall for support.

Harder: Close your eyes while holding the pose.

4. Tree Pose (Vrksasana)

Purpose: Enhances balance and strengthens the legs.

Step-by-Step Instructions:

Starting Position: Stand tall with your feet together and arms at your sides.

Shift Your Weight: Transfer your weight onto your left foot.

Place Your Right Foot: Bend your right knee and place the sole of your right foot against your left inner thigh, calf, or ankle (avoid the knee joint).

Balance and Align: Bring your hands to your heart in prayer position or extend them overhead.

Engage Your Core: Tighten your abdominal muscles to help maintain balance.

Hold the Pose: Focus on a point in front of you and hold the pose for 30 seconds to 1 minute. Repeat on the other side.

Modifications:

Easier: Place your right foot on your left ankle and keep your toes on the ground for balance.

Harder: Close your eyes or extend your arms in different directions.

5. Seated Forward Bend (Paschimottanasana)
Purpose: Stretches the spine, hamstrings, and calves.

Step-by-Step Instructions:

Starting Position: Sit on the floor with your legs extended straight in front of you.
Lengthen Your Spine: Inhale and reach your arms overhead, lengthening your spine.
Fold Forward: Exhale and hinge at your hips, reaching for your feet, shins, or ankles.
Relax Your Head and Neck: Let your head and neck relax as you fold forward.
Hold the Pose: Stay here for 1-2 minutes, breathing deeply.
Modifications:

Easier: Bend your knees slightly or use a strap around your feet to assist with the forward fold.
Harder: Reach your hands beyond your feet and deepen the stretch.
6. Half Moon Pose (Ardha Chandrasana)
Purpose: Enhances balance and strengthens the legs and core.

Step-by-Step Instructions:

Starting Position: Begin in Warrior II with your right foot forward.
Shift Your Weight: Place your right hand on the floor or a block in front of your right foot.
Lift Your Left Leg: Shift your weight onto your right foot and lift your left leg parallel to the floor.
Extend Your Left Arm: Reach your left arm toward the ceiling, stacking your shoulders and hips.
Balance and Align: Look at your left hand or keep your gaze forward.

Hold the Pose: Stay here for 30 seconds to 1 minute, then slowly return to Warrior II and repeat on the other side.
Modifications:

Easier: Use a block under your supporting hand for extra stability.
Harder: Close your eyes while holding the pose or extend your top arm over your head.
By practicing these yoga poses regularly, you can build strength, improve flexibility, and enhance balance over the long term. Remember to listen to your body and modify poses as needed to suit your individual needs and capabilities.

Chapter 18: Comparative Analysis of Yoga with Other Forms of Exercise

Yoga is often compared to other forms of exercise such as strength training, cardiovascular workouts, and flexibility routines. While each exercise modality has its unique benefits, yoga offers a holistic approach that combines elements of all three. This section provides a detailed comparative analysis to help understand the distinct and overlapping advantages of yoga and other forms of exercise.

1. Yoga vs. Strength Training
Focus and Benefits:

Yoga: Primarily uses body weight to build muscle strength through various asanas (postures). It emphasizes balanced muscle development, functional strength, and endurance. Yoga also incorporates flexibility and mental focus, promoting overall well-being.

Strength Training: Typically involves lifting weights or using resistance machines to increase muscle mass and strength. It targets specific muscle groups and is highly effective for hypertrophy and strength gains.

Muscle Engagement:

Yoga: Engages multiple muscle groups simultaneously, fostering functional strength and coordination. Many yoga poses are isometric, requiring muscles to hold static positions, which enhances endurance.

Strength Training: Often isolates muscle groups for targeted growth. Exercises like squats, deadlifts, and bench presses are compound movements but usually require equipment.

Flexibility and Range of Motion:

Yoga: Inherently combines strength with flexibility, improving joint mobility and range of motion. Stretching is an integral part of yoga practice.

Strength Training: May increase strength without necessarily enhancing flexibility. Stretching routines are often recommended alongside strength training to prevent stiffness.

Mental and Emotional Benefits:

Yoga: Integrates mindfulness and breath control, reducing stress and promoting mental clarity and emotional balance.

Strength Training: Can also reduce stress and improve mood, especially through the release of endorphins, but typically lacks a structured mindfulness component.

Risk of Injury:

Yoga: Generally low-impact and gentle on the joints, though improper alignment can lead to injury.
Strength Training: Higher risk of injury, particularly if heavy weights are used without proper form or supervision.
2. Yoga vs. Cardiovascular Exercise
Focus and Benefits:

Yoga: Improves cardiovascular health indirectly through improved circulation, stress reduction, and breathing techniques. Certain styles like Vinyasa or Power Yoga can elevate the heart rate.
Cardiovascular Exercise: Directly enhances heart and lung function through activities like running, cycling, and swimming, which increase the heart rate for sustained periods.
Heart Rate and Endurance:

Yoga: Generally maintains a moderate heart rate, but dynamic styles can offer more intense cardiovascular benefits.
Cardiovascular Exercise: Elevates the heart rate significantly, improving aerobic capacity and endurance.
Caloric Burn:

Yoga: Burns fewer calories compared to high-intensity cardio workouts, but promotes long-term weight management through stress reduction and muscle toning.
Cardiovascular Exercise: High caloric expenditure, making it effective for weight loss and metabolic health.
Impact on the Body:

Yoga: Low-impact, making it suitable for people with joint issues or those seeking gentle exercise.
Cardiovascular Exercise: Can be high-impact (running) or low-impact (swimming), with varying effects on the joints.
Mental and Emotional Benefits:

Yoga: Strong emphasis on mental health, reducing anxiety and depression through mindfulness.
Cardiovascular Exercise: Boosts mental health through endorphin release and stress relief, though usually without a structured mindfulness practice.
3. Yoga vs. Flexibility Routines (Stretching)
Focus and Benefits:

Yoga: Enhances flexibility as part of a holistic practice that includes strength, balance, and mental focus.
Stretching: Focuses exclusively on improving flexibility and range of motion, typically through static and dynamic stretches.
Holistic Approach:

Yoga: Combines stretching with strength, balance, and mindfulness, offering a comprehensive fitness routine.
Stretching: Targets specific muscles to increase flexibility, often used as a warm-up or cool-down in other exercise routines.
Mindfulness and Relaxation:

Yoga: Integrates breath control and meditation, promoting relaxation and mental clarity.
Stretching: Can be relaxing and meditative but usually lacks a structured mindfulness component.
Functional Flexibility:

Yoga: Improves functional flexibility that enhances everyday movements and posture.
Stretching: Focuses on increasing the flexibility of specific muscles, which can aid in preventing injuries and improving performance in other sports or activities.
Suitability for All Ages and Fitness Levels:

Yoga: Adaptable to various fitness levels and ages, providing modifications for different abilities.
Stretching: Generally accessible to all but may need to be tailored to individual flexibility levels.
Summary and Conclusion
Combining Modalities:

Optimal Fitness: Incorporating yoga with strength training, cardiovascular exercise, and stretching provides a well-rounded fitness routine. This combination ensures comprehensive physical conditioning, mental well-being, and overall health.
Yoga's Unique Position:

Holistic Benefits: Yoga stands out for its holistic approach, offering physical, mental, and emotional benefits. It enhances strength, flexibility, and balance while promoting mindfulness and stress reduction.
Complementary Exercise: While yoga can be a standalone practice, it also complements other forms of exercise by improving flexibility, reducing the risk of injury, and enhancing mental focus.
Individual Preferences and Goals:

Personalization: The best exercise routine depends on individual preferences, goals, and physical conditions. Yoga's adaptability makes it suitable for a wide range of people, whether they seek relaxation, physical fitness, or mental clarity.
By understanding the comparative benefits of yoga and other forms of exercise, individuals can make informed decisions about their fitness routines and choose the practices that best meet their needs and goals.

Chapter 19: Safety and Injury Prevention in Yoga Practice

Yoga is widely regarded as a safe and effective way to improve physical and mental health. However, like any form of physical activity, it carries potential risks if not practiced correctly. Ensuring safety and preventing injury in yoga requires attention to proper technique, body awareness, and mindful practice. This section outlines expert advice on how to practice yoga safely and avoid common injuries.

1. Understanding Your Body
Listen to Your Body:

Awareness: Pay close attention to how your body feels during each pose. Discomfort is normal, but sharp pain or persistent discomfort is a sign to stop.

Modifications: Use modifications and props to adapt poses to your current level of flexibility and strength.

Know Your Limits:

Gradual Progression: Increase the intensity and complexity of poses gradually. Avoid pushing your body into poses that feel beyond your capability.

Individual Differences: Understand that everyone's body is different. What works for one person might not work for another.

2. Proper Technique and Alignment

Learn the Basics:

Foundation: Focus on mastering basic poses and proper alignment before progressing to advanced poses. This builds a strong foundation and reduces the risk of injury.

Instructions: Follow detailed instructions from qualified instructors, whether in-person or via reputable online sources.

Alignment Cues:

Feet and Ankles: Ensure proper placement of feet and grounding through the ankles to maintain stability.

Knees: Avoid hyperextending or locking your knees. Keep a slight bend if needed.

Hips: Align hips squarely in poses to prevent strain on the lower back and hips.

Spine: Maintain a neutral spine. Avoid rounding or over-arching the back.

Shoulders: Keep shoulders relaxed and away from the ears to avoid tension.

3. Using Props and Modifications

Props:

Blocks: Provide support and bring the floor closer, especially in standing poses and forward bends.
Straps: Help achieve a deeper stretch or maintain proper alignment without overreaching.
Bolsters: Offer support and comfort in seated and reclining poses.
Modifications:

Adjusting Poses: Modify poses to suit your flexibility, strength, and any existing injuries. For example, bending the knees in forward folds if hamstrings are tight.
Alternate Poses: Use alternate poses that achieve similar benefits without causing strain.
4. Warm-Up and Cool-Down
Warm-Up:

Dynamic Stretches: Begin with gentle dynamic stretches to increase blood flow and warm up muscles.
Joint Mobility: Include movements that mobilize joints, such as wrist circles, shoulder rolls, and ankle rotations.
Cool-Down:

Static Stretches: Finish with static stretches to help muscles relax and lengthen after the practice.
Breathing Exercises: Incorporate deep breathing exercises to promote relaxation and recovery.
5. Breathing Techniques
Breath Awareness:

Controlled Breathing: Maintain steady, controlled breaths throughout your practice. Avoid holding your breath.
Synchronization: Synchronize your movements with your breath. Inhale during expansions and exhale during contractions.
Avoiding Breath-Holding:

Relaxation: Focus on breathing smoothly and evenly. Breath-holding can lead to tension and reduce oxygen flow to muscles.
6. Progression and Intensity
Gradual Progression:

Incremental Steps: Progress slowly and steadily, allowing your body to adapt to new poses and increased intensity.
Building Strength: Incorporate strength-building poses to support flexibility and reduce the risk of overstretching.
Avoid Overexertion:

Mindful Practice: Avoid pushing your body to the point of exhaustion or pain. Rest when needed.
Balanced Routine: Incorporate a balanced mix of different yoga styles and intensities to prevent overuse injuries.
7. Rest and Recovery
Importance of Rest:

Rest Days: Schedule regular rest days to allow your body to recover and rebuild strength.
Sleep: Ensure adequate sleep to support muscle recovery and overall health.
Injury Management:

Immediate Care: If you experience pain or injury, stop practicing and seek medical advice.
Rehabilitation: Follow appropriate rehabilitation exercises and modifications to prevent further injury and support healing.
8. Seeking Professional Guidance
Qualified Instructors:

Certification: Choose instructors with recognized certifications and experience.

Personalized Attention: Opt for classes that offer personalized attention, especially if you have specific health concerns or injuries.
Medical Advice:

Pre-Existing Conditions: Consult with a healthcare provider before starting yoga, especially if you have pre-existing medical conditions or injuries.
Professional Assessment: Seek professional assessment if you experience persistent pain or discomfort during or after yoga practice.
Conclusion
Practicing yoga safely requires a mindful approach, proper technique, and an understanding of your body's limitations. By incorporating these expert guidelines, you can minimize the risk of injury and maximize the physical and mental benefits of yoga. Remember, yoga is a journey, and the focus should always be on gradual progress, self-awareness, and enjoyment.

Chapter 20: Common Yoga Injuries and Prevention

Yoga is a beneficial practice for physical and mental well-being, but like any physical activity, it carries the risk of injury if not practiced correctly. This chapter will discuss common yoga injuries, their causes, and how to prevent them through proper technique, awareness, and safe practice habits.

Common Yoga Injuries
Wrist Injuries

Cause: Overuse or improper alignment in weight-bearing poses like Downward-Facing Dog or Plank Pose.
Prevention:
Alignment: Ensure wrists are aligned under shoulders in poses. Distribute weight evenly across the hands, pressing into the fingers and the base of the palms.
Strength and Flexibility: Build wrist strength gradually and incorporate wrist stretches into your routine.
Modifications: Use fists or forearms instead of palms for weight-bearing poses to reduce strain.
Shoulder Injuries

Cause: Overextension or improper alignment in poses like Chaturanga Dandasana or inversions.
Prevention:
Alignment: Keep shoulders away from ears, and avoid collapsing into the shoulder joints. Engage shoulder muscles for stability.
Strength and Flexibility: Strengthen shoulder muscles with specific exercises and stretch them regularly to maintain flexibility.
Gradual Progression: Avoid jumping into advanced poses without building sufficient shoulder strength and flexibility.
Lower Back Injuries

Cause: Overarching the back in poses like Upward-Facing Dog or improper alignment in forward bends.
Prevention:
Core Engagement: Engage core muscles to support the lower back in all poses.
Alignment: Maintain a neutral spine in backbends and avoid rounding the back excessively in forward bends.
Modifications: Use props like blocks or straps to assist in maintaining proper alignment and reduce strain.
Knee Injuries

Cause: Improper alignment or excessive pressure in poses like Warrior I/II or Lotus Pose.
Prevention:
Alignment: Ensure the knee is aligned with the ankle in standing poses and avoid deep knee bends if not adequately supported.
Strength and Flexibility: Strengthen surrounding muscles (quadriceps, hamstrings) and improve hip flexibility to reduce knee strain.
Modifications: Use props like blocks under the knee or avoid deep knee bends if experiencing discomfort.
Hamstring Injuries

Cause: Overstretching in forward bends or splits.
Prevention:
Warm-Up: Ensure muscles are warmed up before engaging in deep stretches.
Gradual Progression: Increase flexibility gradually, avoiding forcing the body into deep stretches prematurely.
Proper Technique: Keep a slight bend in the knees in forward bends to protect the hamstrings and lower back.
Neck Injuries

Cause: Poor alignment or excessive strain in poses like Shoulder Stand or Headstand.
Prevention:
Alignment: Keep the neck in a neutral position and avoid excessive tilting or turning.
Support: Use blankets or other props to support the neck in inversions.
Strength and Flexibility: Build neck strength gradually and avoid poses that cause neck strain.
General Prevention Tips
Proper Warm-Up and Cool-Down

Warm-Up: Always start with a gentle warm-up to prepare muscles and joints for the practice.
Cool-Down: End with a cool-down to help muscles relax and recover.
Mindful Practice

Body Awareness: Pay attention to how your body feels in each pose. Avoid pushing into pain or discomfort.
Breathing: Use breath to guide movements, ensuring you are not holding your breath or creating unnecessary tension.
Use of Props

Support: Utilize props such as blocks, straps, bolsters, and blankets to support your practice and maintain proper alignment.
Adaptation: Adjust poses using props to accommodate your body's needs and limitations.
Technique and Alignment

Instruction: Follow detailed instructions from qualified instructors, ensuring you understand proper alignment and technique.
Self-Correction: Use mirrors or videos to check your alignment and make necessary adjustments.
Gradual Progression

Patience: Progress slowly and avoid rushing into advanced poses without adequate preparation.
Building Strength and Flexibility: Work on building overall strength and flexibility gradually to support more challenging poses.
Rest and Recovery

Rest Days: Incorporate rest days into your routine to allow your body to recover.

Listening to Your Body: Take breaks when needed and modify or skip poses if you feel pain or excessive fatigue.
Seeking Professional Guidance

Qualified Instructors: Choose instructors with recognized certifications and experience.
Medical Advice: Consult with healthcare providers before starting yoga, especially if you have pre-existing conditions or injuries.
Conclusion
By understanding common yoga injuries and implementing these prevention strategies, you can enjoy a safe and effective yoga practice. Remember that yoga is a journey of self-discovery and improvement, and maintaining safety is key to a sustainable and fulfilling practice.

Chapter 21: Identifying High-Risk Poses

While yoga can be a safe and beneficial practice for most people, certain poses carry a higher risk of injury, particularly if not performed with proper alignment and body awareness. This chapter identifies some of the high-risk poses in yoga, provides techniques and tips for injury prevention, and emphasizes the importance of proper alignment and body awareness to maintain a safe practice.

High-Risk Poses
Headstand (Sirsasana)

Risk Factors: Neck and cervical spine injuries due to improper weight distribution and lack of neck strength.
Prevention Tips:
Proper Technique: Engage core muscles and lift through the shoulders to avoid putting too much pressure on the neck.
Use of Wall: Practice against a wall for support and balance.
Gradual Progression: Build neck and shoulder strength before attempting a full headstand.
Shoulder Stand (Sarvangasana)

Risk Factors: Neck strain and compression if the body weight is not properly supported.
Prevention Tips:
Alignment: Ensure the neck is in a neutral position, and the weight is supported by the shoulders and upper arms.
Use of Props: Use blankets under the shoulders to maintain proper alignment and reduce neck strain.
Gradual Progression: Build up to the full pose slowly, starting with supported variations.

Plow Pose (Halasana)

Risk Factors: Neck and lower back strain due to deep forward bending and pressure on the cervical spine.
Prevention Tips:
Alignment: Keep the neck long and avoid pressing the chin into the chest.
Use of Props: Place blankets under the shoulders and avoid forcing the feet to the floor.
Gentle Approach: Transition into the pose slowly and listen to your body's limits.
Forward Fold (Uttanasana)

Risk Factors: Hamstring and lower back strain from overstretching.
Prevention Tips:
Bend the Knees: Keep a slight bend in the knees to reduce strain on the hamstrings and lower back.
Engage Core: Engage core muscles to support the lower back.
Use of Props: Use blocks under the hands to reduce the depth of the fold.
Wheel Pose (Urdhva Dhanurasana)

Risk Factors: Lower back and wrist injuries due to deep backbending and weight-bearing on the wrists.
Prevention Tips:
Proper Warm-Up: Warm up thoroughly with gentle backbends and shoulder openers.
Alignment: Ensure proper alignment of the wrists under the shoulders and engage the core and legs.
Gradual Progression: Build strength and flexibility in the back and shoulders before attempting the full pose.
Pigeon Pose (Eka Pada Rajakapotasana)

Risk Factors: Knee and hip injuries from improper alignment and overstretching.

Prevention Tips:
Alignment: Keep the front knee at a comfortable angle and avoid forcing the hips down.
Use of Props: Place a blanket or block under the hip for support.
Gentle Approach: Ease into the pose slowly and avoid pushing into discomfort.
Twisting Poses (e.g., Revolved Triangle Pose)

Risk Factors: Spine and lower back injuries from improper twisting.
Prevention Tips:
Alignment: Lengthen the spine before twisting and initiate the twist from the thoracic spine.
Engage Core: Use core muscles to support the twist and avoid forcing the movement.
Gradual Progression: Increase the depth of the twist gradually and mindfully.
Techniques and Tips for Injury Prevention
Warm-Up and Cool-Down

Importance: Proper warm-up prepares the body for more intense poses, and cool-down aids in muscle recovery.
Techniques: Include dynamic stretches, gentle yoga flows, and breath awareness in the warm-up. Use static stretches and relaxation poses in the cool-down.
Proper Alignment

Focus: Correct alignment is crucial to avoid strain and injury.
Techniques:
Use of Mirrors: Practice in front of a mirror to check alignment.
Instruction: Follow detailed instructions from a qualified teacher.
Proprioception: Develop body awareness through practice and mindful adjustments.

Body Awareness

Listening to Your Body: Pay attention to sensations in the body. Discomfort is normal, but sharp pain is a warning sign.
Mindfulness: Practice mindfulness to stay present and aware of your body's limits.
Breath: Use breath as a guide; if breathing becomes strained, it's a sign to ease back.
Use of Props and Modifications

Props: Use blocks, straps, blankets, and bolsters to support the body and maintain alignment.
Modifications: Modify poses to suit your flexibility, strength, and any pre-existing conditions. There's no need to force the body into a pose.
Building Strength and Flexibility Gradually

Progression: Increase the intensity and complexity of poses slowly.
Foundation: Establish a strong foundation in basic poses before advancing to more challenging ones.
Qualified Instruction

Seek Guidance: Learn from certified yoga instructors who can provide personalized adjustments and corrections.
Workshops and Classes: Attend workshops and classes to deepen your understanding of proper techniques and alignment.
Rest and Recovery

Rest Days: Incorporate rest days into your routine to allow muscles to recover.
Recovery Practices: Use restorative yoga, gentle stretching, and adequate sleep for recovery.
Conclusion

Identifying high-risk poses and practicing them with caution, proper alignment, and body awareness is essential to prevent injuries in yoga. By following these techniques and tips, you can enjoy the benefits of yoga safely and sustainably. Remember, yoga is a practice of mindfulness and balance, both on and off the mat.

Chapter 22: Safe Yoga Practice

Yoga is not just about the poses; it's about how you approach them with mindfulness and care. This chapter focuses on the importance of a safe yoga practice, including effective warm-up and cool-down routines, and the crucial skill of listening to your body.

Warm-Up Routines
Purpose: A warm-up prepares your body physically and mentally for yoga practice, reducing the risk of injury and enhancing performance.

Dynamic Movements

Benefits: Increase blood flow to muscles, improve flexibility, and warm up joints.
Examples: Gentle joint rotations (neck, shoulders, wrists, hips, knees, ankles), spinal movements (cat-cow stretches), and dynamic stretches (leg swings, arm circles).
Sun Salutations (Surya Namaskar)

Purpose: Sequential movements that integrate breath with movement, warming up major muscle groups and joints.
Flow: Begin with a slower pace, gradually increasing speed and intensity with each round.
Breath Awareness

Technique: Practice pranayama (breathing exercises) to deepen breath capacity and focus the mind.
Examples: Deep belly breathing (diaphragmatic breathing), alternate nostril breathing (Nadi Shodhana), or Kapalabhati (skull-shining breath).
Importance of Listening to Your Body
Body Awareness:

Mindful Approach: Pay attention to physical sensations, thoughts, and emotions without judgment.
Self-Regulation: Adjust your practice based on how you feel in the moment.
Signs to Watch For:

Pain vs. Discomfort: Distinguish between sharp pain (indicating potential injury) and discomfort (sensations of stretching or muscle engagement).
Breath Quality: Maintain smooth and controlled breathing; avoid holding your breath or gasping.
Fatigue: Recognize signs of fatigue or overexertion; rest when needed to prevent injury.
Cool-Down Routines
Purpose: Promote relaxation, flexibility, and recovery after physical exertion.

Static Stretches

Technique: Hold stretches for 20-30 seconds, focusing on major muscle groups used during practice.
Examples: Forward bends, hip openers, spinal twists, and gentle backbends.
Restorative Poses

Purpose: Support relaxation and release tension accumulated during practice.
Examples: Child's Pose (Balasana), Legs-Up-the-Wall Pose (Viparita Karani), Corpse Pose (Savasana).
Breath and Meditation

Integration: Use breath awareness and meditation techniques to calm the mind and enhance relaxation.
Focus: Direct attention inward, observing thoughts and sensations without attachment.

Safe Practice Tips
Alignment and Props

Use of Props: Support alignment and modify poses as needed with blocks, straps, blankets, or bolsters.
Mindful Alignment: Maintain proper alignment to prevent strain on joints and muscles.
Gradual Progression

Build Foundation: Master basic poses before advancing to more complex variations.
Listen to Limits: Respect your body's current abilities and avoid pushing beyond comfortable limits.
Hydration and Nutrition

Hydration: Drink water before and after practice to stay hydrated.
Nutrition: Eat a light meal or snack 1-2 hours before yoga; avoid heavy meals that may cause discomfort during practice.
Rest and Recovery

Rest Days: Schedule regular rest days to allow muscles time to recover and repair.
Sleep: Ensure adequate sleep to support physical and mental well-being.
Conclusion
A safe yoga practice begins with mindful preparation, attentive practice, and thoughtful recovery. By incorporating effective warm-up and cool-down routines, listening to your body's signals, and practicing with proper alignment and awareness, you can cultivate a sustainable and fulfilling yoga practice that promotes health and well-being on all levels. Remember, each yoga session is an opportunity to connect with yourself and honor your body's needs.

Chapter 23: Expert Advice from Physiotherapists and Yoga Instructors

Incorporating insights from both physiotherapists and experienced yoga instructors provides a holistic perspective on maintaining a safe and effective yoga practice. This chapter compiles expert advice, combining therapeutic knowledge from physiotherapists with the practical wisdom of yoga instructors, to enhance understanding and application in yoga.

Physiotherapist's Insights
Understanding Movement Patterns

Biomechanics: Emphasize proper alignment and movement patterns to prevent strain and injury.
Individual Assessment: Tailor yoga practice to accommodate individual differences in flexibility, strength, and injury history.
Functional Movement: Integrate yoga poses that support daily activities and promote joint health.
Injury Prevention Strategies

Preventive Techniques: Focus on strengthening stabilizing muscles around joints to enhance stability and reduce injury risk.
Flexibility Training: Incorporate dynamic and static stretching to improve range of motion and muscle elasticity.
Education: Educate practitioners on signs of overuse, proper warm-up techniques, and the importance of gradual progression.

Rehabilitation and Recovery

Therapeutic Approach: Recommend yoga as part of rehabilitation programs to improve mobility, strength, and proprioception.
Progressive Adaptation: Modify poses and sequences to accommodate injuries or post-surgical rehabilitation.
Cross-Disciplinary Collaboration: Advocate for collaboration between physiotherapists and yoga instructors to optimize patient outcomes.
Yoga Instructor's Perspective
Mindful Practice and Awareness

Body Awareness: Cultivate mindfulness to deepen awareness of body alignment, breath, and sensations.
Breath-Centered Movement: Coordinate breath with movement to enhance focus, relaxation, and energy flow.
Intuitive Adjustments: Provide personalized guidance and adjustments to meet individual needs during practice.
Safe and Inclusive Teaching

Instructional Clarity: Offer clear instructions and demonstrations to ensure proper alignment and technique.
Adaptation and Modification: Encourage the use of props and modifications to accommodate varying levels of experience and physical abilities.
Empowerment: Foster a non-judgmental environment that empowers practitioners to honor their bodies and practice self-care.
Holistic Health Benefits

Stress Management: Highlight yoga's role in reducing stress, enhancing mental clarity, and promoting emotional well-being.
Physical Fitness: Emphasize the development of strength, flexibility, and balance through a balanced yoga practice.

Lifestyle Integration: Advocate for the integration of yoga principles into daily life for sustained health benefits beyond the mat.

Collaboration and Integration

Interdisciplinary Approach

Shared Knowledge: Bridge insights from physiotherapy and yoga to optimize physical health and injury prevention strategies.

Continuing Education: Encourage ongoing learning and professional development among both physiotherapists and yoga instructors.

Client-Centered Care: Prioritize the well-being and individual needs of clients through collaborative care planning.

Community and Support

Networking: Facilitate networking opportunities between physiotherapists, yoga instructors, and other healthcare professionals to exchange knowledge and resources.

Peer Support: Foster a supportive community where professionals can share best practices, challenges, and successes in integrating yoga into therapeutic settings.

Conclusion

By integrating expert advice from physiotherapists and yoga instructors, practitioners can cultivate a safe, inclusive, and beneficial yoga practice. Through a balanced approach that emphasizes alignment, mindful movement, injury prevention strategies, and collaborative care, individuals can experience the transformative benefits of yoga while maintaining optimal physical health and well-being. This chapter serves as a resource for both practitioners and professionals seeking to enhance their understanding and application of yoga as a therapeutic modality.

Chapter 24: Yoga for Special Populations - Yoga for Pregnant Women

Yoga offers numerous benefits for pregnant women, promoting physical health, mental well-being, and preparation for childbirth. This chapter focuses on the benefits, precautions, recommended poses with modifications, and postnatal yoga practices tailored for pregnant women.

Benefits of Yoga for Pregnant Women
Physical Health Benefits

Strength and Flexibility: Promotes muscle tone, flexibility, and endurance, which can help support the physical changes during pregnancy and prepare for childbirth.
Balance: Enhances balance and stability as the body's center of gravity shifts.
Pain Relief: Alleviates common pregnancy discomforts such as back pain, sciatica, and swelling.
Breathing: Encourages deep breathing techniques that can be beneficial during labor and delivery.
Mental and Emotional Well-Being

Stress Reduction: Reduces stress, anxiety, and promotes relaxation through mindful movement and breathing exercises.
Mind-Body Connection: Enhances body awareness and fosters a connection with the growing baby.
Sleep Improvement: Promotes better sleep patterns and relaxation.
Precautions for Pregnant Women Practicing Yoga

Consultation with Healthcare Provider

Medical Clearance: Obtain approval from a healthcare provider before starting or continuing a yoga practice during pregnancy, especially if there are pre-existing medical conditions or complications.
Avoiding Overexertion

Moderation: Practice yoga poses and sequences at a comfortable pace, avoiding excessive strain or intensity.
Avoid Supine Positions: After the first trimester, avoid lying on the back for extended periods to prevent compression of the vena cava vein.
Awareness of Body Changes

Listen to Your Body: Modify poses as needed to accommodate physical changes and sensations.
Avoid Overheating: Practice in a well-ventilated space and stay hydrated.
Recommended Poses and Modifications
Gentle Standing Poses

Benefits: Enhance circulation, strengthen leg muscles, and improve balance.
Examples: Tree Pose (Vrksasana), Warrior II (Virabhadrasana II), and Modified Triangle Pose (Trikonasana).
Pelvic Floor Exercises

Benefits: Strengthen pelvic floor muscles to support childbirth and postpartum recovery.
Examples: Kegel exercises, Cat-Cow stretches, and Pelvic Tilts.
Seated and Restorative Poses

Benefits: Promote relaxation, alleviate tension, and improve posture.

Examples: Seated Forward Bend (Paschimottanasana), Butterfly Pose (Baddha Konasana), and Supported Child's Pose (Balasana).
Breathing Techniques (Pranayama)

Benefits: Enhance relaxation, reduce stress, and prepare for labor.
Examples: Deep belly breathing (diaphragmatic breathing), Ujjayi breath (Victorious breath), and Alternate Nostril Breathing (Nadi Shodhana).
Postnatal Yoga Practices
Recovery and Healing

Gentle Movements: Gradually reintroduce yoga postures to aid in physical recovery after childbirth.
Pelvic Floor Exercises: Continue exercises to strengthen pelvic floor muscles and support bladder control.
Bonding and Relaxation

Mother-Baby Bonding: Incorporate gentle movements and soothing techniques to foster bonding with the baby.
Restorative Poses: Support relaxation and stress reduction for new mothers adjusting to postnatal changes.
Supportive Community

Postnatal Yoga Classes: Join specialized classes or groups that cater to postnatal yoga to connect with other new mothers.
Peer Support: Share experiences and receive guidance from instructors knowledgeable in postnatal yoga practices.
Conclusion

Yoga during pregnancy offers significant benefits for physical health, mental well-being, and preparation for childbirth. By practicing yoga safely with modifications and under the guidance of qualified instructors, pregnant women can experience the transformative benefits of yoga while supporting their overall health and preparing for the journey of motherhood. This chapter serves as a resource for integrating yoga into prenatal and postnatal care, emphasizing safety, mindfulness, and the promotion of holistic well-being for expectant mothers.

Chapter 25: Yoga for the Elderly

Yoga offers valuable benefits for the elderly, addressing common age-related issues, promoting physical health, and enhancing overall well-being. This chapter explores gentle yoga practices, chair yoga adaptations, and includes success stories and testimonials illustrating the positive impact of yoga on older adults.

Addressing Common Age-Related Issues
Mobility and Flexibility

Benefits: Improves joint mobility, flexibility, and range of motion.
Poses: Gentle stretches and movements to promote suppleness and ease stiffness.
Balance and Stability

Benefits: Enhances balance, coordination, and reduces the risk of falls.
Poses: Standing poses with support, chair yoga sequences focusing on stability.
Strength and Muscle Tone

Benefits: Maintains muscle strength and supports functional movements.
Poses: Modified versions of standing poses, seated poses with resistance bands or light weights.
Mental Well-Being

Benefits: Reduces stress, promotes relaxation, and enhances mental clarity.
Practices: Mindfulness techniques, breathwork (pranayama), and meditation.
Gentle Yoga Practices and Chair Yoga

Gentle Yoga

Approach: Slow-paced, accessible movements tailored to individual needs.
Poses: Seated and reclining poses, gentle stretches, and guided relaxation techniques.
Chair Yoga

Adaptation: Yoga poses modified to be performed while seated or using a chair for support.
Benefits: Increases accessibility, improves posture, and provides stability for older adults with limited mobility.
Success Stories and Testimonials
Improved Mobility and Pain Relief

Case Study: Mary, 72, experienced reduced joint pain and increased flexibility after regular chair yoga sessions. She now moves with greater ease and enjoys daily activities without discomfort.
Enhanced Balance and Confidence

Testimonial: John, 80, credits chair yoga for improving his balance and confidence in walking. He feels more stable and secure navigating his home and community.
Emotional Well-Being and Stress Reduction

Success Story: Sarah, 68, found chair yoga beneficial for managing stress and anxiety. The mindfulness practices helped her stay calm and centered during challenging times.
Incorporating Yoga into Daily Life

Group Classes: Encourage participation in local senior centers, community centers, or online yoga classes designed for seniors.
Social Connection: Foster a sense of community and camaraderie through group yoga sessions.

Conclusion
Yoga is a valuable tool for promoting physical health, enhancing mobility, and supporting mental well-being among older adults. By adapting yoga practices to suit the needs and abilities of elderly individuals, whether through gentle yoga practices or chair yoga, seniors can experience improved quality of life and a greater sense of vitality. This chapter highlights the transformative benefits of yoga for the elderly, celebrating success stories and testimonials that illustrate the positive impact of yoga on aging gracefully and with resilience.

Chapter 26: Yoga for Individuals with Disabilities

Yoga can be adapted to accommodate individuals with disabilities, promoting physical, mental, and emotional well-being in an inclusive and supportive environment. This chapter explores adaptive yoga techniques, the importance of inclusivity in yoga practice, and resources/support networks available for individuals with disabilities.

Adaptive Yoga Techniques
Customization of Poses

Individualized Approach: Modify traditional yoga poses to suit the specific needs and abilities of individuals with disabilities.
Props and Support: Use props such as blocks, straps, chairs, or bolsters to facilitate safe and comfortable practice.
Seated and Supported Poses

Chair Yoga: Adapt yoga poses to be performed while seated, using a chair for stability and support.
Wall Support: Utilize walls for balance and as a support aid during standing poses.
Mindfulness and Breathwork

Accessible Techniques: Incorporate breathing exercises (pranayama) and mindfulness practices that can be practiced in various positions.
Relaxation: Guide participants through guided relaxation techniques to promote stress reduction and mental clarity.
Inclusivity in Yoga Practice
Creating Accessible Spaces

Physical Environment: Ensure yoga spaces are wheelchair accessible and considerate of different mobility needs.
Communication: Use inclusive language and provide clear instructions that are easy to understand.
Adaptive Instruction

Knowledge and Training: Educate yoga instructors and practitioners on adaptive techniques and considerations for working with individuals with disabilities.
Personalization: Offer personalized modifications and adjustments based on individual capabilities and preferences.
Promoting Participation and Empowerment

Encouragement: Foster a supportive and non-judgmental atmosphere that encourages individuals of all abilities to participate.
Celebrating Progress: Recognize and celebrate achievements, no matter how small, to build confidence and motivation.
Resources and Support Networks
Local Community Centers and Organizations

Yoga Programs: Seek out community centers or yoga studios that offer specialized classes for individuals with disabilities.
Support Groups: Join local support groups or organizations that promote inclusive yoga practices and provide resources.
Online Resources and Apps

Accessible Classes: Access online yoga classes designed specifically for individuals with disabilities, often offering modifications and adaptive techniques.
Educational Materials: Find instructional videos, articles, and guidelines on adaptive yoga practices and inclusivity in yoga.
Professional Networks and Workshops

Continuing Education: Attend workshops, seminars, or training sessions focused on adaptive yoga and disability awareness.

Networking: Connect with professionals in the field, including yoga instructors, physical therapists, and healthcare providers, to exchange knowledge and best practices.

Conclusion

Adaptive yoga practices empower individuals with disabilities to experience the physical, mental, and emotional benefits of yoga in a safe and inclusive environment. By promoting accessibility, providing adaptive techniques, and fostering supportive communities, yoga can become a transformative tool for enhancing overall well-being and quality of life. This chapter emphasizes the importance of inclusivity in yoga practice and highlights resources and support networks available to facilitate participation and empowerment for individuals with disabilities.

Chapter 27: Scientific Research and Limitations - Current State of Yoga Research

Yoga has gained attention in scientific research for its potential health benefits across various domains. This chapter provides an overview of key scientific studies on yoga, discusses limitations and gaps in the research, and explores future directions for advancing yoga research.

Overview of Key Scientific Studies on Yoga
Physical Health Benefits

Cardiovascular Health: Studies indicate yoga's potential to reduce blood pressure, improve heart rate variability, and enhance cardiac function.
Musculoskeletal Health: Research explores yoga's role in improving flexibility, muscle strength, and reducing musculoskeletal pain, particularly in conditions like lower back pain and arthritis.
Respiratory Function: Yoga practices, including pranayama, have been studied for their impact on respiratory health, such as increasing lung capacity and improving breathing efficiency.
Mental and Emotional Well-Being

Stress Reduction: Numerous studies demonstrate yoga's effectiveness in reducing perceived stress levels, cortisol levels, and promoting relaxation responses through mindfulness practices.

Anxiety and Depression: Research suggests yoga may alleviate symptoms of anxiety and depression, potentially through its effects on neurotransmitter levels and stress regulation pathways.

Cognitive Function: Preliminary studies explore yoga's influence on cognitive function, including attention, memory, and executive function, though more research is needed.

Quality of Life and Wellness

Quality of Life: Yoga interventions have shown promise in enhancing overall quality of life metrics, including physical functioning, emotional well-being, and social relationships.

Sleep Quality: Yoga practices are investigated for their potential to improve sleep patterns and alleviate insomnia symptoms, promoting better sleep quality and duration.

Limitations and Gaps in the Research

Methodological Challenges

Study Designs: Many studies are small-scale or lack rigorous controls, limiting the generalizability and reliability of findings.

Long-Term Effects: Longitudinal studies assessing the sustained effects of yoga over extended periods are relatively scarce.

Diversity and Inclusivity

Participant Diversity: Research often lacks diversity in terms of age, gender, ethnicity, and socioeconomic backgrounds, limiting the applicability of findings to broader populations.

Adaptations for Special Populations: More research is needed on the efficacy of yoga for specific populations, such as individuals with disabilities or chronic health conditions.

Mechanistic Understanding

Biological Mechanisms: While some studies explore physiological mechanisms underlying yoga's effects, further research is needed to elucidate the precise biological pathways involved.

Psychological Mechanisms: Understanding how yoga influences psychological processes, such as stress response, emotion regulation, and cognitive function, requires more comprehensive investigation.

Future Directions for Yoga Research

Large-Scale Randomized Controlled Trials (RCTs)

Efficacy and Effectiveness: Conduct more RCTs with larger sample sizes and diverse populations to establish the efficacy and effectiveness of yoga interventions across various health outcomes.

Longitudinal Studies

Sustainability of Effects: Investigate the long-term benefits of regular yoga practice on physical health, mental well-being, and quality of life outcomes.

Mechanistic Studies

Biological Pathways: Explore the underlying biological mechanisms through which yoga exerts its effects, including neurophysiological, immune, and endocrine pathways.

Psychological Mechanisms: Examine how yoga practices influence psychological processes, such as stress resilience, emotion regulation, and cognitive function.

Special Populations and Adaptations

Inclusivity: Focus on adapting yoga practices for diverse populations, including older adults, individuals with disabilities, and those managing chronic health conditions.

Tailored Interventions: Develop and validate yoga interventions tailored to specific health conditions, considering individualized needs and preferences.

Conclusion
Scientific research on yoga continues to expand, highlighting its potential as a holistic approach to enhancing health and well-being. While existing studies demonstrate promising results across physical, mental, and emotional domains, addressing methodological limitations, increasing diversity in participant samples, and exploring mechanistic pathways are critical for advancing the field. Future research efforts should prioritize rigorous study designs, longitudinal assessments, and interdisciplinary collaborations to further elucidate the benefits of yoga and optimize its application in promoting health across diverse populations.

Chapter 28: Critical Analysis of Yoga Myths

Yoga, rooted in ancient tradition, often carries myths and misconceptions that can misguide practitioners and enthusiasts. This chapter aims to debunk common myths, promote evidence-based yoga practices, and provide guidelines for discerning credible yoga information.

Debunking Common Myths and Misconceptions
Myth: Yoga is Only for the Flexible

Reality: Yoga is inclusive and adaptable to all body types and abilities. It focuses on gradual improvement of flexibility, strength, and balance through practice.
Myth: Yoga is Just Stretching

Reality: Yoga encompasses a variety of practices beyond stretching, including breathwork (pranayama), meditation, strength-building poses, and philosophical teachings.
Myth: Yoga is Only for Women

Reality: Yoga is practiced by people of all genders. Historical origins may have cultural contexts, but modern yoga is accessible to everyone.
Myth: You Have to Be Spiritual or Religious to Practice Yoga

Reality: While yoga has spiritual roots, it can be practiced as a secular discipline focused on physical health, mental well-being, and stress reduction.
Myth: Yoga is Too Slow to Provide Cardiovascular Benefits

Reality: Certain yoga styles, such as Vinyasa or Power Yoga, incorporate dynamic movements and sequences that can elevate heart rate and provide cardiovascular conditioning.
Evidence-Based Yoga Practices
Research-Supported Benefits

Physical Health: Improved flexibility, strength, balance, and cardiovascular fitness.
Mental Health: Reduced stress, anxiety, depression, and enhanced mood.
Medical Conditions: Supportive evidence for managing conditions like hypertension, chronic pain, and insomnia.
Recommended Practices

Asana (Physical Postures): Incorporate a balanced mix of poses that target flexibility, strength, and relaxation.
Pranayama (Breathwork): Utilize various breathing techniques to calm the mind, increase focus, and manage stress.
Meditation and Mindfulness: Foster mental clarity, emotional resilience, and a sense of inner peace.
How to Discern Credible Yoga Information
Sources of Information

Qualified Instructors: Seek guidance from certified yoga teachers with reputable training and experience.
Research Publications: Consult peer-reviewed journals and reputable scientific studies for evidence-based information.
Yoga Organizations: Refer to established yoga organizations and associations that uphold standards of practice and education.
Critical Evaluation

Claims and Promises: Be cautious of exaggerated claims or quick-fix solutions related to yoga practices.

Personal Experience: Trust your own experience and listen to your body's responses during yoga practice.

Community Feedback: Engage with fellow practitioners and seek balanced perspectives on different yoga approaches and teachings.

Continued Learning

Continuing Education: Stay informed through workshops, seminars, and continuing education programs that provide updated knowledge and practices.

Openness to Evolution: Recognize that yoga evolves over time, incorporating new research findings and adapting to diverse cultural and global contexts.

Conclusion

Understanding and debunking myths surrounding yoga is essential for fostering a well-informed and effective practice. By embracing evidence-based practices, recognizing the diversity of yoga applications, and critically evaluating sources of information, practitioners can cultivate a meaningful and sustainable yoga journey. This chapter encourages a balanced approach to yoga, grounded in both tradition and contemporary understanding, to maximize its benefits for physical, mental, and emotional well-being.

Chapter 29: Integrating Yoga with Holistic Health - Yoga and Nutrition

Integrating yoga with holistic health involves considering nutrition as a foundational element in supporting yoga practice. This chapter explores the role of diet in yoga, integrates Ayurvedic principles with modern nutrition insights, and provides recipes and meal plans tailored for yogis.

The Role of Diet in Supporting Yoga Practice
Energy and Vitality

Balanced Nutrition: Provides essential nutrients that support physical energy, mental clarity, and overall vitality needed for yoga practice.
Hydration: Emphasizes adequate hydration to maintain fluid balance and support detoxification processes.
Digestive Health

Ayurvedic Perspective: Views digestion as central to overall health, emphasizing mindful eating practices and foods that support digestive efficiency.
Fiber-Rich Foods: Incorporates fruits, vegetables, whole grains, and legumes to promote gastrointestinal health and regularity.
Mind-Body Connection

Food as Fuel: Recognizes food choices that enhance mood stability, mental focus, and emotional well-being, aligning with yoga's holistic approach to mind-body integration.
Ayurvedic Principles and Modern Nutrition
Dosha Balancing

Individualized Nutrition: Considers individual constitutions (doshas) – Vata, Pitta, and Kapha – to determine optimal dietary choices that promote balance and harmony.
Ayurvedic Guidelines: Suggests warming spices (e.g., ginger, turmeric) for digestion, cooling foods (e.g., cucumber, coconut) to pacify heat, and grounding foods (e.g., root vegetables) for stability.
Seasonal Eating

Harmony with Nature: Encourages eating seasonal, locally sourced foods to align with environmental rhythms and support overall well-being.
Adaptability: Adapts dietary choices based on seasonal changes to maintain balance and optimize health throughout the year.
Recipes and Meal Plans for Yogis
Energizing Breakfast Options

Smoothie Bowls: Blend fruits, leafy greens, protein-rich ingredients like nuts or seeds, and superfoods such as chia seeds or acai for sustained energy.
Oatmeal Variations: Prepare oats with plant-based milk, top with fresh fruits, nuts, and a drizzle of honey or maple syrup for added nutrients.
Nourishing Lunch and Dinner Ideas

Buddha Bowls: Combine quinoa or brown rice with roasted vegetables, chickpeas or tofu, avocado, and a tahini or lemon-garlic dressing for a balanced meal.

Vegetarian/Vegan Entrees: Prepare dishes like lentil curry, stir-fried tempeh with vegetables, or stuffed bell peppers with quinoa and black beans.
Snacks and Hydration

Nutrient-Rich Snacks: Opt for hummus with raw veggies, trail mix with nuts and dried fruits, or yogurt with granola for quick energy boosts.
Hydration: Infuse water with cucumber, mint, or lemon to stay hydrated throughout the day, complementing yoga's emphasis on cleansing and rejuvenation.
Conclusion
Integrating yoga with holistic health involves recognizing the interconnectedness of diet, physical practice, and mental well-being. By embracing nutrition as a supportive element in yoga practice, incorporating Ayurvedic principles, and exploring diverse recipes and meal plans, yogis can enhance their overall health, vitality, and harmony with themselves and their environment. This chapter encourages a mindful approach to food choices, emphasizing nourishment, balance, and sustainability in alignment with the principles of yoga and holistic wellness.

Chapter 30: Yoga and Meditation

Yoga and meditation share a profound synergy, enhancing physical, mental, and spiritual well-being through complementary practices. This chapter explores the integration of meditation into yoga practice, highlights techniques for cultivating mindfulness, and discusses the benefits of combining these practices.

The Synergy Between Yoga and Mindfulness
Mind-Body Connection

Yoga as Preparation: Yoga postures (asanas) prepare the body by releasing tension, increasing flexibility, and enhancing physical awareness, facilitating a deeper meditation practice. Mindfulness in Action: Yoga cultivates present-moment awareness, anchoring the mind in the body and breath, which serves as a foundation for meditation.
Breath Awareness

Pranayama Practices: Incorporate breathwork techniques (pranayama) to regulate and deepen the breath, promoting relaxation, focus, and inner stillness conducive to meditation. Integration with Asanas: Coordinate breath with movement during yoga poses to synchronize body and mind, fostering a meditative state of flow.
Inner Exploration

Self-Reflection: Yoga encourages introspection and self-awareness, preparing the mind for meditation by quieting external distractions and turning inward.
Emotional Resilience: Combined practices nurture emotional resilience, enhancing the ability to observe thoughts and emotions without attachment or judgment.
Techniques for Integrating Meditation into Yoga Practice
Mindful Movement

Flow Sequences: Engage in fluid, continuous movements (e.g., Vinyasa flow) that synchronize breath with movement, promoting a meditative flow state.
Conscious Transitions: Emphasize mindful transitions between poses, maintaining awareness of sensations, alignment, and breath throughout the practice.
Seated Meditation

Post-Asana Integration: Transition from physical poses to seated meditation, maintaining body awareness and a calm, focused mind.
Guided Meditation: Use guided meditation sessions or visualization techniques to deepen relaxation and concentration during seated practice.
Mantra Meditation

Chanting Practices: Incorporate Sanskrit mantras or affirmations (e.g., "Om," "So Hum") during yoga and meditation sessions to focus the mind and elevate consciousness.
Repetitive Chants: Repeat mantras silently or aloud, syncing rhythmically with breath cycles to cultivate a meditative state and vibrational harmony.
Benefits of Combined Practices
Stress Reduction and Relaxation

Synergistic Effects: Yoga and meditation together amplify stress-relieving benefits, promoting relaxation responses, and reducing physiological markers of stress (e.g., cortisol levels).
Enhanced Mental Clarity

Focus and Concentration: Integrated practices improve mental focus, sharpening attentional skills and enhancing cognitive function.
Mindful Awareness: Cultivate present-moment awareness and heightened sensory perception, fostering clarity of thought and intuitive insight.
Holistic Well-Being

Emotional Balance: Combined practices nurture emotional resilience, promoting a balanced perspective and adaptive coping strategies.
Spiritual Growth: Deepen spiritual connection and inner peace, transcending the physical realm to explore higher states of consciousness and self-realization.
Conclusion
Yoga and meditation form a powerful union, synergizing physical movement with mindfulness practices to promote holistic well-being. By integrating meditation techniques into yoga practice, practitioners can enhance their ability to cultivate inner peace, resilience, and mental clarity. This chapter underscores the transformative potential of combined yoga and meditation practices, inviting individuals to explore and deepen their journey toward physical, mental, and spiritual harmony through intentional practice and mindful presence.

Chapter 31: Yoga and Traditional Medical Treatments

Yoga has increasingly been recognized as a complementary approach to traditional medical treatments, supporting overall health and well-being through integrative practices. This chapter explores the synergy between yoga and conventional medicine, highlighting their complementary roles in enhancing health outcomes.

Complementary Approaches to Health
Integration with Conventional Medicine

Holistic Care: Emphasizes a holistic approach to health, integrating yoga practices with conventional medical treatments to address physical, mental, and emotional aspects of well-being.
Collaborative Care: Encourages collaboration between healthcare providers, yoga instructors, and practitioners to optimize patient care and treatment outcomes.
Supportive Role in Chronic Conditions

Chronic Pain Management: Yoga offers gentle movements, stretches, and relaxation techniques that may alleviate chronic pain symptoms and improve quality of life.
Cardiovascular Health: Complements medical interventions for heart disease by promoting stress reduction, improving cardiovascular function, and supporting lifestyle changes.

Mental Health and Emotional Well-Being

Anxiety and Depression: Integrates mindfulness practices, breathwork, and meditation to augment psychotherapeutic interventions for managing anxiety, depression, and related disorders.
Stress Management: Enhances stress resilience, reduces cortisol levels, and fosters relaxation responses, which can benefit overall mental health and emotional balance.
Evidence-Based Benefits
Physical Health

Musculoskeletal Benefits: Improves flexibility, muscle strength, and joint mobility, which may aid in rehabilitation and physical therapy.
Respiratory Function: Enhances lung capacity and efficiency through pranayama techniques, supporting respiratory health and pulmonary rehabilitation.
Psychological Well-Being

Cognitive Function: Promotes cognitive vitality and executive function through mindfulness practices and focused attention training.
Sleep Quality: Facilitates relaxation and stress reduction, improving sleep patterns and supporting sleep hygiene practices.
Patient Empowerment and Self-Care

Empowering Patients: Encourages active participation in self-care through yoga practice, fostering a sense of empowerment and personal responsibility for health outcomes.
Health Education: Provides educational resources on yoga's therapeutic benefits, promoting informed decision-making and lifestyle modifications.
Practical Applications and Case Studies
Integrative Treatment Plans

Personalized Approach: Tailors yoga practices to individual health needs and treatment goals, integrating them into comprehensive care plans.

Progress Monitoring: Evaluates progress through objective measures and patient-reported outcomes, assessing the impact of yoga on health outcomes.

Case Studies and Success Stories

Pain Management: Illustrates how yoga interventions have supported pain relief and functional improvement in patients with chronic pain conditions.

Mental Health: Highlights cases where yoga has contributed to reducing symptoms of anxiety, depression, and enhancing overall emotional well-being.

Conclusion

Yoga's integration with traditional medical treatments offers a holistic framework for promoting health and healing. By recognizing and utilizing yoga's therapeutic benefits alongside conventional medicine, practitioners can enhance patient care, improve treatment outcomes, and empower individuals to actively engage in their well-being journey. This chapter emphasizes the importance of collaborative healthcare approaches, evidence-based practices, and patient-centered care in harnessing the potential of yoga as a complementary modality for holistic health and wellness.

Chapter 32: Exploring Different Styles of Yoga - Comparative Overview of Yoga Styles

Yoga encompasses a diverse array of styles, each offering unique characteristics, benefits, and approaches to practice. This chapter provides a comparative overview of major yoga styles, guides readers in choosing the right style based on goals and preferences, and explores transitioning between styles for a personalized yoga journey.

Characteristics and Benefits of Major Yoga Styles
Hatha Yoga

Foundation: Focuses on physical postures (asanas) and breath control (pranayama) to achieve balance between body and mind.
Benefits: Improves flexibility, strength, and overall body awareness. Promotes relaxation and stress reduction through gentle movements and mindful breathing.
Vinyasa Yoga

Dynamic Flow: Emphasizes fluid, synchronized movements with breath (vinyasa), transitioning between poses in a continuous sequence.
Benefits: Enhances cardiovascular fitness, builds muscular endurance, and cultivates mindfulness through rhythmic movement and breath coordination.

Iyengar Yoga

Alignment Focus: Prioritizes precise alignment of postures using props (e.g., blocks, straps) to support correct positioning and enhance stability.
Benefits: Develops strength, flexibility, and body awareness. Suitable for individuals seeking therapeutic benefits or precise technique refinement.
Ashtanga Yoga

Structured Sequence: Follows a set series of poses (asanas) in a progressive sequence, linked with synchronized breath (vinyasa).
Benefits: Builds physical strength, endurance, and stamina. Promotes internal heat generation for detoxification and purification of the body.
Bikram (Hot) Yoga

Heated Environment: Practices a specific sequence of 26 poses and two breathing exercises in a room heated to approximately 40°C (104°F).
Benefits: Enhances flexibility, promotes detoxification through sweating, and may improve circulation and cardiovascular health. Requires tolerance to heat and hydration.
Kundalini Yoga

Energetic Activation: Integrates dynamic movements, breathwork (pranayama), chanting (mantra), and meditation to awaken spiritual energy (kundalini).
Benefits: Cultivates self-awareness, emotional balance, and spiritual growth. Focuses on energy flow and inner transformation through holistic practices.
Restorative Yoga

Relaxation and Healing: Utilizes props (e.g., bolsters, blankets) to support passive poses held for extended durations, promoting deep relaxation and stress relief.
Benefits: Facilitates physical and mental relaxation, enhances recovery from injury or illness, and rejuvenates the body's natural healing processes.
Choosing the Right Style for Your Goals and Preferences
Consider Personal Objectives

Physical Goals: Identify whether you seek to improve flexibility, strength, cardiovascular fitness, or relaxation.
Mental Goals: Determine if you prioritize stress reduction, mindfulness development, emotional balance, or spiritual exploration.
Assess Experience Level

Beginner-Friendly Styles: Start with styles like Hatha, Iyengar, or Restorative Yoga for foundational learning and technique refinement.
Intermediate to Advanced Styles: Progress to dynamic styles such as Vinyasa, Ashtanga, or Kundalini Yoga as strength, flexibility, and familiarity with yoga principles develop.
Explore Preferences

Environment: Consider preferences for heated rooms (Bikram), quiet meditation (Kundalini), precise alignment (Iyengar), or flowing sequences (Vinyasa).
Holistic Approach: Choose styles that resonate with your holistic health goals, incorporating physical, mental, and spiritual dimensions of well-being.
Transitioning Between Styles
Gradual Progression

Build Foundation: Begin with foundational styles and gradually explore more challenging or dynamic practices as proficiency and comfort levels increase.

Incorporate Variety: Integrate elements from different styles (e.g., restorative poses after a vigorous Vinyasa session) to balance intensity and promote recovery.
Listen to Your Body

Adaptation and Adjustment: Pay attention to how your body responds to different styles, modifying intensity or duration as needed to prevent injury and optimize benefits.
Consult Instructors: Seek guidance from qualified instructors or experienced practitioners when transitioning between styles to ensure safe and effective practice.
Mindful Exploration

Reflect and Refine: Reflect on experiences with different styles, noting preferences, challenges, and improvements in physical and mental well-being.
Continued Learning: Maintain curiosity and openness to explore new styles, adapting your practice over time to align with evolving goals and aspirations.
Conclusion
Exploring different styles of yoga offers a pathway to discovering practices that resonate with individual preferences, goals, and holistic health needs. By understanding the characteristics, benefits, and considerations of major yoga styles, practitioners can tailor their yoga journey to cultivate physical strength, mental clarity, emotional balance, and spiritual growth. This chapter encourages an exploratory and adaptable approach to yoga practice, fostering a lifelong journey of self-discovery, well-being, and personal transformation through diverse and enriching yoga experiences.

Chapter 33: Deep Dive into Specific Styles

This chapter delves into specific yoga styles, exploring their unique characteristics, practices, and benefits. Each style offers distinct approaches to physical postures, breathwork, and mental focus, contributing to holistic well-being and personal growth.

Hatha Yoga: Foundation and Practice
Foundation:

Rooted in Tradition: Hatha yoga integrates physical postures (asanas), breath control (pranayama), and meditation to balance body and mind.
Gentle Approach: Emphasizes slower-paced movements and longer-held poses to cultivate strength, flexibility, and inner awareness.
Practice:

Asana Variations: Includes a wide range of poses from basic to advanced, focusing on alignment and mindful movement.
Breath Awareness: Incorporates pranayama techniques to synchronize breath with movement, promoting relaxation and concentration.
Benefits:

Physical Health: Improves flexibility, muscular strength, and posture alignment.
Mental Well-Being: Reduces stress, enhances mental clarity, and fosters a sense of inner calm and balance.
Vinyasa Flow: Movement and Breath
Movement and Flow:

Dynamic Sequences: Links breath with continuous movement through a series of poses (asanas), creating a fluid and rhythmic practice.
Creative Expression: Allows for variations in sequencing and pace, promoting creativity and spontaneity in practice.
Breath Integration:

Breath Coordination: Emphasizes Ujjayi pranayama (victorious breath) to regulate breath throughout the practice, generating internal heat and energy.
Flow State: Facilitates a meditative flow state, enhancing focus, mindfulness, and mind-body connection.
Benefits:

Cardiovascular Fitness: Increases heart rate and circulation, improving cardiovascular health and endurance.
Stress Reduction: Promotes relaxation, releases tension, and cultivates mental clarity and emotional balance.
Ashtanga Yoga: Discipline and Sequence
Discipline and Structure:

Traditional Approach: Follows a specific sequence of poses (asanas) linked with synchronized breath (vinyasa), progressing through primary, intermediate, and advanced series.
Self-Practice: Encourages a disciplined daily practice (Mysore style) with individualized guidance from a teacher.
Sequence and Progression:

Systematic Progression: Builds strength, flexibility, and stamina systematically, challenging practitioners to advance at their own pace.
Focused Attention: Cultivates concentration, mindfulness, and perseverance through consistent practice and adherence to the sequence.
Benefits:

Physical Endurance: Enhances physical fitness, muscular endurance, and stamina through rigorous and structured practice.
Mental Discipline: Develops mental focus, resilience, and self-discipline, fostering a balanced and integrated approach to life.
Yin Yoga: Stretch and Surrender
Stretch and Release:

Passive Poses: Involves long-held, passive poses (asanas) typically held for 3-5 minutes or longer, targeting deep connective tissues and joints.
Mindful Relaxation: Emphasizes relaxation and surrender, allowing gravity to deepen stretches and release muscular tension.
Therapeutic Approach:

Stimulates Meridians: Influences the body's energy flow (chi or prana) through targeted stretching of meridian lines, promoting energetic balance and healing.
Mind-Body Awareness: Cultivates introspection, mindfulness, and acceptance of present sensations and emotions.
Benefits:

Joint Health: Improves flexibility and mobility, especially in hips, pelvis, and spine.

Stress Relief: Induces deep relaxation, reduces chronic stress, and supports emotional well-being through surrendering into poses.
Restorative Yoga: Healing and Relaxation
Healing and Support:

Supported Poses: Utilizes props (blankets, bolsters, blocks) to fully support the body in gentle, passive poses, promoting deep relaxation and healing.
Nurturing Environment: Creates a safe and nurturing space for relaxation, rejuvenation, and restoration of the body's natural equilibrium.
Mindful Relaxation:

Extended Holds: Encourages longer holds (5-20 minutes) in each pose to facilitate profound relaxation, release tension, and calm the nervous system.
Breath Awareness: Integrates conscious breathing techniques (pranayama) to deepen relaxation and enhance inner awareness.
Benefits:

Stress Reduction: Promotes deep relaxation, reduces cortisol levels, and supports the parasympathetic nervous system's response (rest and digest).
Recovery and Renewal: Facilitates recovery from fatigue, illness, or injury, enhancing overall well-being and resilience.
Conclusion

Each yoga style offers a unique pathway to physical health, mental clarity, and emotional well-being, catering to diverse preferences and goals. By exploring and understanding these styles—Hatha, Vinyasa Flow, Ashtanga, Yin, and Restorative—practitioners can cultivate a balanced yoga practice that aligns with their individual needs, preferences, and aspirations for holistic growth and self-discovery. This chapter encourages readers to explore these styles mindfully, embracing their transformative potential to enhance overall health and enrich life's journey through dedicated and intentional yoga practice.

Chapter 34: Cultural and Historical Context of Yoga - The Origins of Yoga

Yoga, an ancient practice with deep historical and cultural roots, has evolved over millennia, shaping its philosophical foundations, practices, and global influence. This chapter explores the historical development, cultural significance, and influence of ancient texts and teachings that have shaped yoga into the diverse and transformative discipline known today.

Historical Development and Evolution
Early Origins:

Indus Valley Civilization: Traces roots to the ancient Indus Valley civilization (2600-1900 BCE), where early forms of yoga and meditation were depicted in seals and artifacts.
Vedic Period: Emerged from Vedic traditions (1500-500 BCE), integrating spiritual practices, rituals, and hymns focused on cosmic harmony and individual enlightenment.
Classical Yoga Systems:

Pre-Classical Yoga: Explored in early Upanishads (800-200 BCE), emphasizing inner contemplation, meditation, and philosophical inquiry into the nature of reality and self.
Classical Yoga: Codified by Patanjali's Yoga Sutras (200 BCE - 200 CE), outlining the Eight Limbs of Yoga (Ashtanga Yoga) as a systematic path to spiritual liberation (moksha).
Medieval and Post-Classical Periods:

Bhakti and Tantra Yoga: Flourished during the medieval era (500-1500 CE), emphasizing devotion (bhakti) to a personal deity and esoteric practices (tantra) for spiritual transformation.
Hatha Yoga: Emerged in the post-classical period (900-1500 CE), focusing on physical purification techniques (asanas, pranayama) to prepare the body for spiritual practices.
Cultural Significance of Traditional Practices
Spiritual and Philosophical Foundations:

Dharma and Karma: Upholds principles of dharma (ethical duty) and karma (law of cause and effect), guiding moral conduct and actions in alignment with cosmic order (Rta).
Samsara and Moksha: Addresses the cyclical nature of existence (samsara) and liberation (moksha), seeking freedom from worldly attachments through self-realization and union with the divine (yoga).
Yogic Traditions and Lineages:

Guru-Disciple Tradition: Reveres spiritual teachers (gurus) and lineage (parampara) transmission, preserving oral teachings, practices, and spiritual insights through generations.

Rituals and Festivals: Celebrates yoga's cultural heritage through rituals, festivals (e.g., Guru Purnima), and pilgrimage sites (e.g., Rishikesh, Varanasi) as sacred spaces for spiritual practice and reflection.

Influence of Ancient Texts and Teachings

Yoga Sutras of Patanjali:

Eight Limbs of Yoga: Explores ethical principles (yamas, niyamas), physical postures (asanas), breath control (pranayama), concentration (dharana), meditation (dhyana), and absorption (samadhi).

Guidance for Practice: Provides a philosophical framework and practical guidance for cultivating self-discipline, mental clarity, and spiritual awakening.

Bhagavad Gita:

Yoga of Action (Karma Yoga): Expounds on the path of selfless action, duty (dharma), and devotion (bhakti), emphasizing detachment from outcomes and dedication to higher principles.

Integral Yoga: Integrates karma yoga, bhakti yoga (devotion), jnana yoga (knowledge), and raja yoga (meditation) as paths to spiritual realization and union with the divine.

Hatha Yoga Pradipika and Gheranda Samhita:

Physical Purification: Details techniques for cleansing (shatkarmas), physical postures (asanas), energy control (pranayama), and spiritual practices (mudras, bandhas) to awaken latent energies (kundalini) and achieve physical and spiritual balance.

Conclusion

The origins of yoga reflect a rich tapestry of spiritual inquiry, cultural expression, and philosophical exploration that continues to resonate across diverse global communities today. By understanding its historical development, cultural significance, and foundational texts, practitioners can deepen their appreciation for yoga's transformative potential and timeless wisdom. This chapter invites readers to explore yoga not only as a physical practice but as a profound journey of self-discovery, spiritual growth, and alignment with universal truths that transcend time and culture.

Chapter 35: Modern Yoga Practices

Yoga, rooted in ancient traditions, has undergone significant evolution in the contemporary world, adapting to global contexts while preserving its cultural heritage and philosophical essence. This chapter explores how yoga has evolved, the integration of tradition with modernity, and the delicate balance between cultural respect and innovation in shaping modern yoga practices.

Evolution of Yoga in the Contemporary World

Global Popularity and Accessibility:

Western Influence: Gained popularity in the West during the 20th century, influenced by figures like Swami Vivekananda, Paramahansa Yogananda, and yoga pioneers who introduced yoga to Western audiences.
Mainstream Integration: Widely embraced for physical fitness, stress reduction, and holistic well-being, contributing to yoga's global reach and accessibility through studios, gyms, and online platforms.
Diversity of Yoga Styles and Practices:

Emergence of Hybrid Styles: Blends traditional yoga with contemporary fitness trends (e.g., power yoga, hot yoga) to cater to diverse preferences and health goals.
Specialized Applications: Adaptations for therapeutic purposes (e.g., yoga therapy, prenatal yoga) and niche populations (e.g., seniors, athletes) reflect yoga's versatility and applicability in modern lifestyles.
Technological Integration:

Online and Digital Platforms: Facilitates virtual classes, tutorials, and global community engagement, enhancing accessibility and flexibility in yoga practice.
Wearable Technology: Incorporates yoga tracking devices and apps for monitoring performance, progress, and biofeedback during yoga sessions.
Integrating Tradition with Modernity
Preserving Philosophical Roots:

Core Principles: Upholds foundational teachings of yoga sutras, Bhagavad Gita, and classical texts to cultivate ethical values, mindfulness, and spiritual awareness.

Mind-Body Connection: Emphasizes holistic integration of physical postures (asanas), breathwork (pranayama), meditation, and philosophical inquiry into contemporary yoga teachings.
Innovative Teaching Methods:

Educational Approaches: Incorporates evidence-based practices, scientific research, and anatomy studies to enhance teaching methodologies and student learning outcomes.
Adaptive Techniques: Develops modifications, variations, and progressive sequences to accommodate diverse abilities, body types, and health conditions.
Cultural Sensitivity and Adaptation:

Respect for Origins: Acknowledges and honors yoga's cultural roots, Sanskrit terminology, rituals, and traditional practices within modern contexts.
Global Diversity: Celebrates diversity and inclusivity, embracing multicultural perspectives, interpretations, and adaptations of yoga across different societies and belief systems.
Balancing Cultural Respect with Innovation
Ethical Considerations:

Authenticity and Integrity: Ensures accurate representation and transmission of yoga's cultural heritage, avoiding appropriation or commercial exploitation.
Cultural Exchange: Promotes respectful dialogue, collaboration, and mutual learning between traditional practitioners, modern yoga instructors, and global communities.
Community Engagement:

Social Responsibility: Engages in community outreach, charitable initiatives, and yoga service projects to promote social justice, health equity, and well-being for underserved populations.

Environmental Stewardship: Advocates for sustainable practices, eco-consciousness, and mindful consumption in yoga studios, retreat centers, and global yoga events.

Educational Leadership:

Continuing Education: Encourages ongoing learning, professional development, and ethical guidelines for yoga teachers and practitioners to uphold standards of competence, safety, and cultural sensitivity.

Dialogue and Collaboration: Facilitates intercultural exchanges, conferences, and academic research to deepen understanding, foster innovation, and preserve yoga's legacy for future generations.

Conclusion

Modern yoga practices reflect a dynamic synthesis of tradition and innovation, adapting ancient wisdom to contemporary lifestyles and global contexts. By honoring yoga's philosophical roots, embracing diverse expressions of practice, and promoting cultural respect, modern yoga cultivates a transformative journey of self-discovery, holistic well-being, and interconnectedness with the broader community and world. This chapter invites readers to explore the evolving landscape of yoga, celebrating its timeless teachings while embracing opportunities for growth, adaptation, and positive impact in the modern era.

Chapter 36: Advanced Practices for Experienced Yogis - Beyond the Basics

For seasoned practitioners looking to deepen their yoga journey, this chapter explores advanced practices, mastering complex asanas, developing a personal practice, and tips for continuous growth and learning in yoga.

Mastering Advanced Asanas
Progressive Approach:

Building Foundations: Emphasizes mastering foundational poses (asanas) before advancing to more challenging variations.
Incremental Progress: Gradually introduces advanced poses, focusing on alignment, strength, flexibility, and mindful awareness.
Advanced Postures:

Arm Balances: Includes poses like Bakasana (Crow Pose), Astavakrasana (Eight-Angle Pose), and Pincha Mayurasana (Forearm Stand) to develop upper body strength and balance.
Inversions: Explores headstands (Sirsasana), handstands (Adho Mukha Vrksasana), and shoulder stands (Sarvangasana) for cultivating stability, concentration, and overcoming fear.
Backbends and Twists:

Heart Openers: Practices like Urdhva Dhanurasana (Wheel Pose) and Kapotasana (Pigeon Pose) to deepen spinal flexibility, open the chest, and energize the body.
Spinal Twists: Includes Ardha Matsyendrasana (Half Lord of the Fishes Pose) and Marichyasana (Sage Marichi's Pose) to improve spinal mobility, digestion, and detoxification.
Developing a Personal Practice
Self-Reflection and Goal Setting:

Clarifying Intentions: Identifies personal goals, intentions, and areas of focus for the yoga practice (e.g., physical fitness, mental clarity, spiritual growth).
Progress Tracking: Maintains a journal or log to record progress, insights, challenges, and breakthroughs in the practice journey.
Customizing Routine and Sequence:

Tailored Practice: Designs a sequence of asanas, pranayama, meditation, and relaxation techniques that align with individual needs, preferences, and time constraints.
Variety and Adaptation: Incorporates variations, modifications, and props to address specific strengths, weaknesses, and areas for improvement.
Consistency and Discipline:

Daily Commitment: Establishes a consistent daily practice, dedicating time and space for yoga amidst busy schedules and life commitments.
Self-Motivation: Cultivates self-discipline, resilience, and intrinsic motivation to overcome challenges and maintain continuity in practice.
Tips for Continuous Growth and Learning
Seek Guidance and Mentorship:

Experienced Teachers: Enrolls in workshops, retreats, or private sessions with knowledgeable instructors to receive personalized guidance, corrections, and advanced teachings.
Peer Support: Participates in community classes, yoga groups, or online forums to share experiences, insights, and inspiration with fellow practitioners.
Exploration of Yoga Philosophy and Wisdom:

Study of Scriptures: Deepens understanding of yoga philosophy, ethics (yamas and niyamas), and spiritual teachings from classical texts (e.g., Yoga Sutras, Bhagavad Gita).
Integration into Practice: Applies philosophical principles to enhance mindfulness, self-awareness, and alignment with higher spiritual principles in daily life.
Embrace Challenges and Growth Edges:

Mindful Push: Embraces discomfort, challenges, and growth edges in practice to expand physical capabilities, mental resilience, and emotional intelligence.
Progressive Overload: Gradually increases intensity, duration, or complexity of poses and practices to stimulate continuous improvement and adaptation.
Conclusion
Advanced yoga practices offer experienced yogis an opportunity for profound growth, mastery of challenging poses, and deepening spiritual awareness. By developing a personal practice, setting clear intentions, and embracing continuous learning, practitioners can evolve their yoga journey beyond the basics, cultivating resilience, discipline, and inner transformation on and off the mat. This chapter encourages a balanced approach to advanced yoga, integrating physical prowess with spiritual inquiry and holistic well-being for a fulfilling and enriching lifelong practice.

Chapter 37: The Journey of Yoga

Yoga is more than a physical practice; it is a transformative journey that unfolds through self-discovery, mindfulness, and integration of body, mind, and spirit. This chapter explores the profound and personal aspects of the yoga journey, highlighting its stages, challenges, and rewards for practitioners at all levels.

Embarking on the Path
Awakening to Yoga:

Initial Encounter: Begins with curiosity, interest, or a desire for physical fitness, stress relief, or spiritual exploration. Introduction to Practice: Attends a class, workshop, or discovers yoga through books, media, or recommendations, experiencing the benefits of relaxation, flexibility, and inner peace.
Foundations of Practice:

Learning Basics: Focuses on mastering fundamental asanas (poses), breathwork (pranayama), and meditation techniques under the guidance of a teacher or through self-study. Building Consistency: Establishes a regular practice routine to develop physical strength, mental focus, and emotional resilience.
Deepening Commitment
Exploration and Expansion:

Diverse Styles and Techniques: Explores different yoga styles (e.g., Hatha, Vinyasa, Yin) and therapeutic applications (e.g., yoga therapy, prenatal yoga) to meet evolving physical, mental, and emotional needs. Integration of Philosophy: Studies yoga philosophy, ethics, and spiritual principles (e.g., yamas and niyamas) to cultivate mindfulness, compassion, and self-awareness.
Challenges and Growth:

Physical Challenges: Faces physical limitations, injuries, or setbacks, learning resilience and patience through modifications, rest, and gradual progression. Emotional and Mental Exploration: Confronts inner obstacles, fears, or emotional blockages, using yoga as a tool for self-healing, stress management, and emotional balance.
Transformation and Integration
Holistic Well-Being:

Mind-Body Connection: Deepens awareness of the interconnectedness between physical sensations, emotions, and thoughts, fostering holistic well-being and self-care.

Lifestyle Integration: Applies yoga principles off the mat, making conscious choices in nutrition, relationships, and daily routines that align with values of mindfulness, sustainability, and inner harmony.

Spiritual Inquiry:

Inner Journey: Explores deeper layers of consciousness, spirituality, and existential questions through meditation, self-inquiry, and contemplative practices.

Union with Higher Self: Seeks unity (yoga) with the divine, inner peace, and transcendence beyond egoic identity, experiencing moments of clarity, insight, and profound connection.

Sustaining the Practice

Lifelong Dedication:

Continuous Learning: Embraces yoga as a lifelong journey of growth, evolution, and self-discovery, remaining open to new teachings, insights, and transformative experiences.

Community and Support: Engages with a supportive yoga community, attending classes, workshops, or retreats, and contributing to the collective energy of learning and sharing.

Sharing Wisdom:

Teaching and Mentorship: Shares yoga wisdom and experiences with others through teaching, mentoring, or volunteering in yoga outreach programs, fostering inspiration and empowerment in others.

Legacy of Yoga: Cultivates a legacy of peace, compassion, and holistic well-being, inspiring future generations to embrace yoga as a path to health, happiness, and spiritual fulfillment.

Conclusion

The journey of yoga is a profound exploration of self-discovery, transformation, and integration, offering practitioners a path to physical vitality, mental clarity, emotional resilience, and spiritual awakening. By embracing the stages of awakening, deepening commitment, transformation, and sustaining practice, individuals embark on a transformative journey that extends beyond the mat, enriching their lives and contributing to the well-being of the global community. This chapter invites readers to embark on their unique yoga journey, honoring its transformative potential to cultivate inner peace, harmony, and unity with the infinite possibilities of existence.

Chapter 38: Personal stories

Personal stories of advanced yoga practitioners offer profound insights into their transformative journeys, challenges, and profound growth through yoga practice. These narratives often highlight the deeper dimensions of yoga beyond physical postures, illustrating how dedicated practice can impact one's life on multiple levels — physically, mentally, emotionally, and spiritually. Here are some key aspects and themes commonly found in personal stories of advanced practitioners:

Transformation and Growth: Advanced practitioners often share how yoga has transformed their lives, both on and off the mat. They may describe overcoming physical limitations, achieving milestones in challenging poses, and experiencing profound shifts in their mental and emotional well-being.

Spiritual Awakening: Many advanced practitioners speak about their spiritual journey through yoga, describing moments of clarity, insight, and connection to a higher consciousness or divine presence. They may share experiences of inner peace, spiritual growth, and a deeper sense of purpose in life.

Challenges and Resilience: Personal stories often include accounts of challenges faced along the yoga journey—such as injuries, setbacks, or moments of self-doubt—and how these obstacles were overcome through perseverance, patience, and a commitment to the practice.

Integration into Daily Life: Advanced practitioners frequently discuss how they integrate yoga principles—such as mindfulness, compassion, and self-awareness—into their daily routines and interactions. They may share practical tips for maintaining balance, managing stress, and living in alignment with their values.

Community and Support: Many stories highlight the importance of community and support networks within the yoga community. Advanced practitioners often acknowledge the role of teachers, mentors, and fellow practitioners in their growth and development, as well as the joy of sharing their journey with others.

Teaching and Sharing Wisdom: Some advanced practitioners choose to become yoga teachers or mentors themselves, inspired to share their wisdom and experiences with others. They may discuss the fulfillment they find in teaching, guiding students, and contributing to the broader yoga community.

Lifelong Journey: Lastly, personal stories often emphasize that yoga is a lifelong journey of continuous learning, exploration, and self-discovery. Advanced practitioners recognize that there is always more to learn and experience, and they remain open to new teachings, challenges, and opportunities for growth.

Overall, personal stories of advanced yoga practitioners serve to inspire, educate, and empower others on their own yoga journeys. They offer insights into the transformative power of yoga and illustrate the profound impact it can have on physical health, mental well-being, and spiritual evolution. These stories celebrate the diversity of experiences within the yoga community and highlight the universal principles of growth, resilience, and self-discovery that unite practitioners around the world.

Chapter 39: The Spiritual and Philosophical Aspects of Yoga

Yoga, beyond its physical practice, encompasses profound spiritual and philosophical dimensions that have guided practitioners for centuries. This chapter delves into the spiritual and philosophical foundations of yoga, exploring its rich heritage, key teachings, and practical applications in contemporary life.

Spiritual Foundations of Yoga
Unity and Connection (Yoga):

Union of Body, Mind, and Spirit: Yoga aspires to unite the individual consciousness with universal consciousness, fostering a sense of interconnectedness and harmony.

Pathways to Liberation: Various paths (yogas) such as karma yoga (path of selfless action), bhakti yoga (path of devotion), jnana yoga (path of knowledge), and raja yoga (path of meditation) offer avenues for spiritual growth and self-realization.

Inner Transformation:

Purification and Self-Discovery: Practices like asanas (postures), pranayama (breath control), and meditation facilitate inner purification, clarity of mind, and heightened awareness.

Evolution of Consciousness: Yoga philosophy emphasizes the journey from ignorance (avidya) to wisdom (vidya), transcending egoic attachments to realize one's true nature (atman) and interconnectedness with the divine (Brahman).

Philosophical Teachings of Yoga

Yamas and Niyamas:

Ethical Principles: Yamas (restraints) and niyamas (observances) provide guidelines for ethical conduct (e.g., non-violence, truthfulness, contentment) and personal discipline (e.g., self-study, surrender to the divine will).

Foundation for Righteous Living: Practicing yamas and niyamas cultivates virtues, integrity, and spiritual maturity, fostering a balanced and harmonious life.

Yoga Sutras of Patanjali:

Eight Limbs of Yoga: Patanjali's classical text outlines a systematic path (Ashtanga Yoga) comprising ethical guidelines (yamas and niyamas), physical postures (asanas), breath control (pranayama), sense withdrawal (pratyahara), concentration (dharana), meditation (dhyana), and absorption (samadhi).

Psychological Insights: Explores the nature of the mind (chitta), fluctuations of consciousness (vrittis), and methods to attain inner stillness, clarity, and transcendental awareness.

Practical Applications in Contemporary Life
Mindfulness and Presence:

Present-Moment Awareness: Yoga encourages mindfulness practices, anchoring awareness in the present moment to reduce stress, enhance focus, and deepen self-awareness. Integration with Daily Activities: Applies yogic principles to work, relationships, and daily routines, promoting conscious living, compassion, and equanimity.
Self-Realization and Liberation:

Journey of Self-Inquiry: Through practices like self-reflection, meditation, and contemplation, individuals explore the nature of the self (atman) and its connection to universal consciousness (Brahman).
Freedom from Suffering: Yoga philosophy addresses the causes of suffering (kleshas), offering pathways to liberation (moksha) from egoic attachments, ignorance, and the cycle of birth and death (samsara).
Contemporary Relevance and Integration
Interfaith Dialogue and Harmony:

Universal Principles: Yoga's inclusive philosophy and spiritual teachings foster interfaith dialogue, mutual respect, and harmony among diverse religious and spiritual traditions.
Global Appeal: Embraced worldwide for its universal principles of unity, compassion, and inner peace, transcending cultural, religious, and geographical boundaries.
Environmental Consciousness:

Yoga and Ecology: Advocates for environmental stewardship, sustainability, and reverence for the interconnectedness of all life forms (ecosystem) through mindful consumption and eco-friendly practices.

Yogic Lifestyle: Promotes simplicity, non-harming (ahimsa), and respect for nature as integral components of a yogic lifestyle rooted in ecological consciousness.
Conclusion
The spiritual and philosophical aspects of yoga offer a profound framework for holistic living, spiritual growth, and inner transformation. By exploring its spiritual foundations, ethical principles, and practical applications in contemporary life, individuals can cultivate mindfulness, compassion, and wisdom, fostering harmony within themselves and the world around them. This chapter invites readers to delve deeper into yoga's timeless teachings, integrating spiritual insights and philosophical wisdom into their personal journey of self-discovery, inner peace, and spiritual fulfillment.

Chapter 40: Creating a Lifelong Yoga Journey

Embarking on a lifelong yoga journey entails cultivating a sustainable and enriching practice that evolves with personal growth and changing life circumstances. This chapter explores essential strategies, principles, and practical tips for individuals committed to integrating yoga into their daily lives for long-term health, well-being, and spiritual development.

Commitment to Consistent Practice
Establishing Routine and Discipline:

Daily Practice: Cultivates a regular yoga routine, dedicating time each day for physical postures (asanas), breathwork (pranayama), meditation, and relaxation.
Adaptability: Adjusts practice based on personal needs, energy levels, and schedules, incorporating shorter sessions during busy periods and longer practices during leisure time.
Setting Intentions and Goals:

Clarity of Purpose: Defines intentions and goals for the yoga journey, whether to enhance physical fitness, reduce stress, deepen spiritual connection, or achieve specific milestones in practice.
Progress Tracking: Maintains a journal or log to monitor progress, reflect on insights, and celebrate achievements along the journey.
Deepening Self-Awareness and Mindfulness
Mind-Body Connection:

Somatic Awareness: Cultivates awareness of bodily sensations, breath patterns, and subtle energy flows during yoga practice, enhancing mindfulness and presence.
Embodied Wisdom: Integrates yoga philosophy and teachings into daily life, applying principles of non-harming (ahimsa), moderation (brahmacharya), and self-study (svadhyaya) in relationships, work, and self-care.
Exploring Meditation and Contemplative Practices:

Mindful Meditation: Incorporates meditation techniques (e.g., mindfulness meditation, loving-kindness meditation) to quiet the mind, cultivate inner stillness, and deepen spiritual inquiry.
Contemplative Practices: Engages in self-inquiry, reflection on philosophical texts (e.g., Yoga Sutras, Bhagavad Gita), and dialogue with mentors or spiritual guides to deepen understanding and insight.
Integrating Yoga into Lifestyle and Relationships

Yoga Off the Mat:

Daily Mindfulness: Applies yoga principles (e.g., compassion, gratitude) in daily interactions, decision-making, and responses to challenges, fostering emotional resilience and harmony.
Holistic Health Practices: Adopts a balanced lifestyle that includes nutritious diet choices, adequate sleep, regular physical activity, and stress management techniques aligned with yogic principles.
Community and Support Networks:

Sangha (Community): Engages with like-minded individuals in yoga classes, workshops, retreats, or online forums to share experiences, insights, and mutual support.
Mentorship and Guidance: Seeks guidance from experienced yoga teachers, mentors, or spiritual leaders for personalized advice, encouragement, and inspiration on the path of yoga.
Embracing Lifelong Learning and Growth
Continuing Education and Exploration:

Diverse Yoga Styles: Explores various yoga styles (e.g., Hatha, Vinyasa, Yin) and specialized practices (e.g., yoga therapy, prenatal yoga) to broaden knowledge, skills, and experience in yoga.
Workshops and Retreats: Participates in workshops, seminars, or residential retreats to deepen understanding of specific aspects of yoga (e.g., meditation retreats, philosophical studies).
Adaptation and Evolution:

Aging Gracefully: Adapts yoga practice to accommodate changing physical abilities, health conditions, and life stages (e.g., pregnancy, postnatal recovery, senior years), emphasizing safety, self-care, and holistic well-being.

Innovation and Creativity: Embraces creativity in practice, exploring new poses, sequences, and therapeutic approaches to maintain enthusiasm and adaptability in long-term yoga practice.

Cultivating a Spiritual Legacy

Service and Contribution:

Yoga Outreach: Volunteers in community service projects, outreach programs, or yoga initiatives that promote accessibility, inclusivity, and well-being for underserved populations.

Teaching and Mentorship: Shares yoga wisdom and experiences with others through teaching, mentoring, or leadership roles in yoga communities, inspiring others on their own paths of self-discovery and growth.

Legacy of Wisdom and Compassion:

Living Yoga Principles: Embodies the principles of yoga in daily life as a beacon of wisdom, compassion, and integrity, leaving a positive impact on family, friends, and the broader community.

Generational Transmission: Passes on teachings, values, and practices of yoga to future generations, nurturing a legacy of holistic health, spiritual fulfillment, and interconnectedness with the universe.

Conclusion

Creating a lifelong yoga journey involves dedication, mindfulness, and a commitment to growth and self-discovery. By integrating yoga into daily life, nurturing self-awareness, embracing community support, and fostering continuous learning, individuals embark on a transformative path of holistic health, spiritual awakening, and inner peace. This chapter encourages readers to cultivate a sustainable yoga practice that evolves with their lives, fostering resilience, joy, and a profound connection to the timeless wisdom of yoga.

Conclusion: Summarizing Key Takeaways

Throughout this comprehensive exploration of yoga's multifaceted dimensions, from its physical practices to its spiritual and philosophical depths, several key takeaways emerge. These insights encapsulate the transformative power of yoga and its potential to enrich every aspect of life:

Holistic Well-Being: Yoga offers a holistic approach to health, integrating physical fitness, mental clarity, emotional balance, and spiritual growth. By practicing yoga, individuals cultivate resilience, vitality, and a profound sense of well-being that extends beyond the mat.

Mind-Body Connection: Through mindful movement, breathwork, and meditation, yoga enhances awareness of the mind-body connection. This heightened awareness fosters self-discovery, inner peace, and the ability to navigate life's challenges with equanimity.

Spiritual Exploration: Yoga provides pathways for spiritual inquiry and growth, inviting practitioners to explore deeper dimensions of consciousness, unity with the divine, and the timeless wisdom found in ancient teachings.

Community and Support: Engaging with the yoga community offers invaluable support, camaraderie, and opportunities for shared growth. Whether through classes, workshops, or online forums, the yoga community fosters inspiration, learning, and mutual encouragement.

Lifelong Journey: Yoga is a lifelong journey of continuous learning and evolution. As practitioners deepen their practice over time, they adapt to changing circumstances, embrace new challenges, and cultivate resilience and flexibility — both physically and mentally.

Legacy of Wisdom: By embodying yoga's principles of compassion, mindfulness, and self-awareness in daily life, practitioners leave a positive legacy for future generations. Through teaching, mentoring, and service, they inspire others to embark on their own journeys of self-discovery and well-being.

Global Impact: Yoga transcends cultural boundaries, fostering global unity and understanding through its universal principles of unity, peace, and interconnectedness. As yoga continues to evolve in the modern world, its teachings remain relevant and transformative for individuals and societies alike.

In conclusion, yoga is not merely a practice but a profound philosophy and way of life that empowers individuals to thrive physically, mentally, emotionally, and spiritually. As we integrate yoga into our lives, we embark on a transformative journey of self-discovery, healing, and connection — to ourselves, to others, and to the world around us. May this journey of yoga continue to inspire and uplift, guiding us towards greater harmony, compassion, and fulfillment in every moment.

Encouraging Continuous Exploration and Learning

As you conclude your journey through the depths of yoga, it's essential to embrace a mindset of continuous exploration and learning. Here are some key encouragements to keep in mind:

Embrace Curiosity: Approach yoga with an open heart and a curious mind. Stay curious about different yoga styles, philosophies, and teachings. Each exploration deepens your understanding and enriches your practice.

Stay Open to Growth: Recognize that yoga is a lifelong journey of growth and evolution. Embrace challenges as opportunities for learning and transformation. Allow yourself to grow physically, mentally, emotionally, and spiritually through your practice.

Seek Guidance: Continue to seek guidance from experienced teachers, mentors, and spiritual leaders. Their wisdom and insights can offer new perspectives and help navigate challenges on your yoga journey.

Explore Beyond the Mat: Extend yoga beyond physical postures. Explore meditation, pranayama (breathwork), yoga philosophy, and ethical principles (yamas and niyamas). These aspects deepen your practice and enhance overall well-being.

Integrate into Daily Life: Integrate yoga principles into your daily life. Practice mindfulness, compassion, and gratitude in your interactions with others. Apply yogic teachings to decision-making, relationships, and self-care practices.

Stay Inspired: Stay connected to the yoga community. Attend workshops, retreats, or join online forums to stay inspired and connected with like-minded individuals. Share your experiences and learn from others on similar paths.

Celebrate Progress: Celebrate your progress and achievements along the way. Keep a journal to reflect on insights gained, challenges overcome, and moments of growth. Celebrating milestones keeps you motivated and inspired.

Remain Humble and Patient: Understand that growth in yoga takes time and patience. Be kind to yourself on days when your practice feels challenging or stagnant. Trust in the process and stay committed to your journey.

By encouraging continuous exploration and learning, you enrich your yoga practice and cultivate a deeper connection with yourself and the world around you. Embrace the journey with an open heart, and let the transformative power of yoga unfold in your life every day.

Final Thoughts on the Future of Yoga Practice and Science

As we look ahead to the future of yoga practice and its intersection with scientific inquiry, several exciting developments and possibilities emerge. Here are some final thoughts on what the future may hold:

Integration of Tradition and Innovation: The future of yoga practice will likely see a continued integration of traditional wisdom with modern innovations. This fusion may include advancements in yoga therapy, personalized yoga practices based on individual health data, and the incorporation of technology to enhance accessibility and effectiveness.

Scientific Validation: As interest in yoga's health benefits grows, there will likely be increased scientific research to validate its therapeutic effects. Studies may explore the physiological, psychological, and neurological impacts of yoga, shedding light on its mechanisms of action and optimal practices for various health conditions.

Personalized and Adaptive Practices: With advancements in wearable technology and artificial intelligence, the future of yoga practice may include personalized and adaptive yoga programs. These programs could adjust based on real-time biometric data, individual goals, and feedback, optimizing outcomes and adherence.

Inclusivity and Accessibility: Efforts to make yoga more inclusive and accessible to diverse populations will likely expand. This includes adapting yoga practices for different ages, abilities, and cultural contexts, as well as addressing barriers such as physical limitations and socioeconomic factors.

Global Influence and Cultural Exchange: Yoga's global reach will continue to foster cultural exchange and mutual understanding. As practitioners and teachers from different backgrounds share their knowledge and experiences, yoga's principles of unity, compassion, and peace will resonate across borders.

Ethical Considerations: Discussions on yoga's ethical foundations, such as ahimsa (non-harming) and social responsibility, may gain prominence. This includes addressing issues of cultural appropriation, sustainability in yoga products and practices, and ethical guidelines for teaching and practicing yoga.

Yoga as a Lifestyle: Beyond physical postures, yoga may increasingly be embraced as a holistic lifestyle that integrates mindfulness, ethical living, and spiritual inquiry. This holistic approach promotes overall well-being and supports individuals in navigating the complexities of modern life with clarity and compassion.

Education and Professional Standards: There may be advancements in yoga education and professional standards to ensure quality teaching, ethics, and safety. This includes ongoing training for teachers, certification programs, and standards of practice that uphold yoga's integrity and values.

In conclusion, the future of yoga practice holds promise for continued growth, innovation, and integration with scientific research and technological advancements. As yoga evolves, its timeless principles and transformative potential remain foundational, guiding practitioners toward greater health, harmony, and spiritual fulfillment in an ever-changing world. Embracing these possibilities with openness and respect for yoga's heritage ensures that its benefits are accessible and meaningful to individuals and communities worldwide.

Appendices

Glossary of Yoga Terms

Asana: Physical posture or pose practiced in yoga.

Pranayama: Breath control exercises in yoga.

Dhyana: Meditation; the practice of cultivating focused attention and awareness.

Samadhi: State of meditative absorption, the final stage of Patanjali's Eight Limbs of Yoga.

Yamas: Ethical guidelines in yoga, including non-violence (ahimsa) and truthfulness (satya).

Niyamas: Personal observances in yoga, such as purity (saucha) and self-study (svadhyaya).

Chakra: Energy center in the subtle body, believed to influence physical and emotional well-being.

Mantra: Sacred sound or phrase used in meditation and chanting.

Mudra: Symbolic hand gesture or seal used in meditation and yoga practice.

Prana: Vital life force energy; breath.

Vinyasa: Flowing sequence of yoga poses synchronized with breath.

Hatha Yoga: Classical form of yoga emphasizing physical postures (asanas) and breath control (pranayama).

Kundalini: Coiled energy at the base of the spine; often associated with spiritual awakening.

Om (Aum): Sacred sound and mantra in Hinduism and yoga, symbolizing the universe and consciousness.

Savasana: Corpse pose; relaxation posture practiced at the end of yoga sessions.

Ujjayi: Breath technique in which the practitioner breathes through the nose with a slight constriction in the throat, creating an audible whispering sound.

Yogi/Yogini: Practitioner of yoga (male/female).

Yoga Sutra: Ancient text attributed to Patanjali, outlining the philosophy and practices of yoga.

Namaste: Traditional greeting or salutation, often accompanied by a gesture of bringing the palms together at the heart center.

Sankalpa: Intention or resolve set during yoga practice or meditation.

Sutra: Thread; aphoristic teachings in yoga and Hindu philosophy.

Vedanta: Philosophical system based on the Upanishads, exploring the nature of reality and the self.

Ayurveda: Traditional Indian system of medicine and holistic health practices.

Drishti: Focused gaze or focal point in yoga postures.

Guru: Spiritual teacher or guide.

Japa: Repetition of a mantra or sacred syllable.

Karma: Action; law of cause and effect in Hinduism and Buddhism.

Lila: Divine play; the concept that the universe is a manifestation of divine creativity.

Moksha: Liberation; spiritual liberation or release from the cycle of birth and death (samsara).

Samsara: Cycle of birth, death, and rebirth; the wheel of existence in Hinduism and Buddhism.

Tapas: Austerity; discipline or effort in spiritual practice.

Yoga Nidra: Yogic sleep; a guided relaxation and meditation technique.

Bhakti: Devotion; the path of love and devotion to the divine.

Dharma: Duty, righteousness; cosmic law and order in Hinduism and Buddhism.

Ganesha/Ganesh: Hindu deity with an elephant head, remover of obstacles.

Hanuman: Hindu monkey deity, symbolizing devotion and strength.

Krishna: Hindu deity, avatar of Vishnu, central figure in the Bhagavad Gita.

Lakshmi: Hindu goddess of wealth, prosperity, and abundance.

Shakti: Divine feminine energy and power.

Shiva: Hindu deity, creator and destroyer of the universe; associated with meditation and asceticism.

Vishnu: Hindu deity, preserver and protector of the universe; associated with compassion and devotion.

Yogi tea: Spiced tea blend often enjoyed by yoga practitioners.

Bhagavad Gita: Hindu scripture comprising a conversation between Krishna and Arjuna on duty and righteousness.

Sanskrit: Ancient Indo-Aryan language, sacred language of Hinduism and yoga.

This glossary provides definitions of key terms used in yoga practice and philosophy, enhancing understanding and appreciation of its rich heritage and teachings.

Practical Application:

Integration into Daily Life: Yoga philosophy offers practical principles for living beyond the mat. Readers can integrate mindfulness by practicing present-moment awareness in daily activities, such as eating mindfully or cultivating compassion in interactions with others. Ethical considerations (yamas and niyamas) guide decision-making, promoting honesty (satya), non-violence (ahimsa), and contentment (santosha) in everyday life.

Advanced Practices: Beyond mastering foundational poses (asanas), readers may seek guidance on advancing their practice. This could involve exploring challenging poses (asanas) like inversions or arm balances, deepening pranayama (breathwork) techniques, or engaging in more intensive meditation practices (dhyana).

Personalized Routine: Creating a personalized yoga routine involves aligning practice with individual goals and needs. For physical fitness, sequences can focus on strength, flexibility, or recovery. Emotional well-being may benefit from restorative practices or meditation. Guidance on adapting routines for varying schedules and lifestyles ensures sustainability and relevance.

Spiritual and Philosophical Inquiry:

Deeper Understanding: Readers interested in yoga philosophy may inquire about recommended readings or resources to deepen their understanding. Books on classical yoga texts (Yoga Sutras of Patanjali), Upanishads, or contemporary interpretations provide insights into meditation practices (dhyana), the path of devotion (bhakti), and the quest for self-realization.

Mindfulness and Meditation: Practical guidance on integrating mindfulness and meditation into daily life supports readers in cultivating inner peace and mental clarity. Techniques such as mindful breathing (pranayama), guided visualizations, or mantra meditation help sustain focus and presence amidst daily challenges.

Ethical Considerations: Exploring ethical principles (yamas and niyamas) in depth helps readers apply yoga philosophy ethically. Ahimsa (non-harming) informs compassionate actions, while satya (truthfulness) fosters integrity. Understanding these principles enhances self-awareness and fosters harmony in relationships and communities.

Health and Well-being:

Managing Health Conditions: Yoga's therapeutic benefits extend to managing specific health conditions such as back pain, anxiety, or insomnia. Readers benefit from learning targeted poses (asanas), pranayama (breathwork), and relaxation techniques tailored to alleviate symptoms and promote healing.

Modifications and Adaptations: Addressing modifications for poses ensures inclusivity and safety in practice. Guidance on adapting poses for injuries, physical limitations, or different body types empowers readers to practice yoga safely and effectively, promoting long-term health and well-being.

Holistic Health Practices: Beyond physical poses, holistic health practices include nutrition, stress management, and lifestyle adjustments. Readers explore integrative approaches that complement yoga, such as Ayurvedic principles, mindfulness-based stress reduction (MBSR), or integrative medicine modalities.

Community and Resources:

Finding Qualified Teachers: Identifying reputable yoga teachers, studios, or online platforms aligns with readers' preferences and goals. Recommendations for certification programs, teacher directories, or personal referrals help establish a supportive learning environment and deepen practice.

Connecting with Like-Minded Individuals: Building community through workshops, retreats, or online forums fosters shared learning and inspiration. Networking opportunities enhance personal growth, encourage exploration of diverse perspectives, and cultivate meaningful connections within the yoga community.

Deeper Immersion Experiences: Opportunities for retreats or advanced training programs provide transformative experiences for dedicated practitioners. Immersion in specialized practices (e.g., yoga nidra, yoga therapy) deepens understanding, enhances skills, and nurtures a lifelong commitment to yoga practice and personal growth.

Scientific and Research-Based Insights:

Evidence-Based Benefits: Access to scientific studies validates yoga's benefits for mental health, stress reduction, flexibility, and cardiovascular health. Readers benefit from understanding research findings on physiological and psychological impacts, guiding informed decisions and enhancing confidence in yoga's therapeutic potential.

Navigating Information: Discerning credible sources and evidence-based practices helps readers navigate the wealth of information available. Critical evaluation of research methodologies, expert recommendations, and peer-reviewed publications supports evidence-informed decisions in selecting practices aligned with personal health goals.

Innovations in Yoga Therapy: Emerging trends in yoga therapy, including personalized practices and integrative approaches, provide new avenues for managing health challenges. Awareness of innovative applications (e.g., trauma-sensitive yoga, therapeutic yoga for chronic pain) empowers readers to explore holistic healthcare options and optimize well-being.

Cultural and Global Perspectives:

Respectful Engagement: Respecting yoga's cultural origins while practicing in diverse global contexts promotes cultural awareness and sensitivity. Readers explore cultural narratives, historical contexts, and traditional teachings to deepen understanding and honor yoga's heritage with reverence.

Preservation and Promotion: Contributing to the preservation of yoga's cultural integrity involves supporting cultural initiatives, community collaborations, and educational outreach. Promoting inclusivity, cultural exchange, and mutual respect within the global yoga community fosters unity and collective stewardship of yoga's legacy.

Bridging Cultures: Yoga serves as a bridge between diverse cultural and spiritual traditions, fostering mutual understanding and shared human experience. Readers engage in cross-cultural dialogue, interfaith exploration, and global citizenship to cultivate respect, appreciation, and interconnectedness across boundaries.

Future Directions:

Emerging Trends: Awareness of emerging trends in yoga, such as personalized practices, technological advancements, and sustainability initiatives, informs readers' anticipation of future developments. Insights into evolving practices and innovations inspire exploration, adaptation, and integration of progressive approaches into personal and professional yoga endeavors.

Evolution of Yoga: Yoga's evolution to meet modern societal needs includes promoting mental health, social well-being, and environmental sustainability. Readers envision yoga as a dynamic practice that adapts to contemporary challenges, integrates diverse perspectives, and promotes inclusive wellness strategies.

Ethics and Responsibility: Exploring ethical considerations in yoga practice, including sustainability practices, social responsibility, and ethical guidelines for teaching and practicing yoga, guides readers in embodying yogic values. Commitment to ethical integrity fosters compassionate leadership, environmental stewardship, and collective well-being within the global yoga community.